Atlas of Minimally Invasive Thoracic Surgery (VATS)

Atlas of Minimally Invasive Thoracic Surgery (VATS)

Robert J. McKenna, Jr, MD
Chief, Thoracic Surgery
Program Director, General Thoracic Surgery Fellowship
Surgical Director, Women's Guild Lung Institute
Cedars-Sinai Medical Center
Los Angeles, California

Ali Mahtabifard, MD
Attending Surgeon
Cedars-Sinai Center for Chest Diseases
Associate Director, Thoracic Surgery Residency Program
Cedars-Sinai Medical Center
Los Angeles, California

Scott J. Swanson, MD
Director, Minimally Invasive Thoracic Surgery
Brigham and Women's Hospital
Chief Surgical Officer
Dana-Farber Cancer Institute
Professor of Surgery
Harvard Medical School
Boston, Massachusetts

ELSEVIER
SAUNDERS

ELSEVIER
SAUNDERS

1600 John F. Kennedy Blvd.
Ste 1800
Philadelphia, PA 19103-2899

ATLAS OF MINIMALLY INVASIVE THORACIC SURGERY (VATS)   ISBN: 978-1-4160-6263-9

Notices

Knowledge and best practice in this field are constantly changing. As new research and experience broaden our understanding, changes in research methods, professional practices, or medical treatment may become necessary.

Practitioners and researchers must always rely on their own experience and knowledge in evaluating and using any information, methods, compounds, or experiments described herein. In using such information or methods they should be mindful of their own safety and the safety of others, including parties for whom they have a professional responsibility.

With respect to any drug or pharmaceutical products identified, readers are advised to check the most current information provided (i) on procedures featured or (ii) by the manufacturer of each product to be administered, to verify the recommended dose or formula, the method and duration of administration, and contraindications. It is the responsibility of practitioners, relying on their own experience and knowledge of their patients, to make diagnoses, to determine dosages and the best treatment for each individual patient, and to take all appropriate safety precautions.

To the fullest extent of the law, neither the Publisher nor the authors, contributors, or editors assume any liability for any injury and/or damage to persons or property as a matter of products liability, negligence or otherwise, or from any use or operation of any methods, products, instructions, or ideas contained in the material herein.

Library of Congress Cataloging-in-Publication Data
Mckenna, Robert J. (Robert Joseph), 1951-
  Atlas of minimally invasive thoracic surgery (VATS) / Robert J. Mckenna Jr, Ali Mahtabifard, Scott J. Swanson.–1st ed.
    p. ; cm.
  Includes bibliographical references.
  ISBN 978-1-4160-6263-9 (hardcover : alk. paper) 1. Chest–Endoscopic surgery–Atlases. I. Mahtabifard, Ali. II. Swanson, Scott J. III. Title.
  [DNLM: 1. Thoracic Surgery, Video-Assisted–methods–Atlases. 2. Surgical Procedures, Minimally Invasive–methods–Atlases. 3. Thoracic Surgical Procedures–methods–Atlases. WF 17]
  RD536.M33 2011
  617.5'40597–dc22

                                                                        2010032551

Acquisitions Editor: Judith A. Fletcher
Developmental Editor: Roxanne Halpine Ward
Publishing Services Manager: Anne Altepeter
Team Manager: Radhika Pallamparthy
Project Managers: Cindy Thoms and Vijay Antony Raj Vincent
Designer: Steven Stave

Printed in China

Last digit is the print number: 9 8 7 6 5 4 3 2

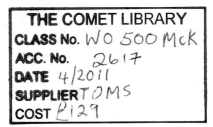

Thanks to my wife and best friend, Kathy, and our children for tolerating my crazy life and for liking me anyway. Also, to my father for showing me how to be a good person, good doctor, and good educator

– Robert J. McKenna, Jr.

To the most important people to me–my beautiful wife, Neda, who is not only the pillar of my life, but also a colleague who shares my love and commitment to medicine and makes it all worthwhile; and to my mother, for whom education and excellence have always been a priority and whose love and sacrifice made it so that I could achieve something meaningful

– Ali Mahtabifard

To my family, who have always understood and been there for support of the rather chaotic life I lead; and in particular to my mother, who quietly set the foundation for all of the great opportunities that I have been incredibly fortunate enough to have

– Scott J. Swanson

CONTRIBUTORS

Cynthia S. Chin, MD
Assistant Professor, Cardiothoracic Surgery
    Mount Sinai School of Medicine
    New York, New York

A. Atiq Durrani, MD
Orthopaedic Spine Surgeon, President
    Center for Advanced Spine Technologies
    Cincinnati, Ohio

Seth D. Force, MD
Associate Professor of Surgery
    Division of Cardiothoracic Surgery
    Emory University
    Atlanta, Georgia

Robert A. Frantz, MD
Assistant Professor of Anesthesiology
    Department of Anesthesiology
    Cedars-Sinai Medical Center
    Los Angeles, California

Kemp H. Kernstine, MD, PhD
Chief, Division of Thoracic Surgery
    Director, Lung Cancer and Thoracic
    Oncology Program
    City of Hope National Medical Center
    Professor, Beckman Research Institute
    Duarte, California

Mark J. Krasna, MD, FACS
Medical Director
    The Cancer Institute
    St. Joseph Medical Center
    Towson, Maryland

Ali Mahtabifard, MD
Attending Surgeon
    Cedars-Sinai Center for Chest Diseases
    Associate Director, Thoracic Surgery
    Residency Program
    Cedars-Sinai Medical Center
    Los Angeles, California

Robert J. McKenna, Jr, MD
Chief, Thoracic Surgery
    Program Director, General Thoracic Surgery
    Fellowship
    Surgical Director, Women's Guild Lung Institute
    Cedars-Sinai Medical Center
    Los Angeles, California

Robert J. McKenna, III, BS, MBS
University of Southern California
    Marshall School of Business
    Tufts University, School of Medicine
    Staff Research Associate I
    Translation Oncology Research, Inc.
    University of California, Los Angeles
    School of Medicine
    Los Angeles, California

Allan Pickens, MD
Assistant Professor of Surgery
    Cardiothoracic Surgery
    Emory University Hospital
    Atlanta, Georgia

Eric W. Schneeberger, MD
Cardiothoracic Surgeon
    Atrial Fibrillation Center
    Deaconess Hospital
    Cincinnati, Ohio

Karen S. Sibert, MD
Associate Professor of Anesthesiology
    Department of Anesthesiology
    Cedars-Sinai Medical Center
    Los Angeles, California

Scott J. Swanson, MD
Director, Minimally Invasive Thoracic Surgery
    Brigham and Women's Hospital
    Chief Surgical Officer
    Dana-Farber Cancer Institute
    Professor of Surgery
    Harvard Medical School
    Boston, Massachusetts

Randall Kevin Wolf, MD
Director
    Cardiothoracic Surgery
    Deaconess Hospital
    Cincinnati, Ohio

James T. Wu, MD
Instructor in Thoracic Surgery
    Department of Surgery
    City of Hope National Medical Center
    Duarte, California

PREFACE

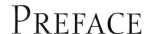

We think that minimally invasive thoracic surgery is good for patients and our specialty. The evidence is now overwhelming that operations that previously required thoracotomy incisions can now be performed safely by video-assisted thoracoscopic surgery (VATS), without compromising the efficacy of the operation. Compared to a thoracotomy, VATS offers patients comparable or reduced morbidity and mortality, earlier return to regular activities, earlier discharge from the hospital, and an overall lower cost. All thoracic surgeons need to understand this and learn the techniques of minimally invasive thoracic surgery, regardless of where they are in their careers, in order to offer these benefits to our patients. The purpose of this atlas is to enable thoracic surgeons to accomplish this transition from open surgery to minimally invasive surgery.

Atlas of Minimally Invasive Thoracic Surgery (VATS) is designed to be a detailed "how to" manual for VATS procedures. The initial chapters present basic concepts of VATS techniques, and the bulk of the remaining chapters focus on step-by-step details of the most commonly performed advanced VATS procedures. Accompanying the book is a DVD with videos of the procedures corresponding to each chapter. The videos are also available on the book's companion website at www.ExpertConsult.com.

We would like to dedicate this book to our patients, who do battle with a very difficult foe and teach us daily about true courage and heroism. Each one of them gives us the inspiration to do better and dedicate ourselves to devising the best therapy possible, hence the development of minimally invasive thoracic surgery.

Robert J. McKenna, Jr, MD
Ali Mahtabifard, MD
Scott J. Swanson, MD

Video Contents on DVD

Video Contents on DVD; also available on www.expertconsult.com

CONTENTS

SECTION

I

General Topics

CHAPTER 1

GENERAL SETUP AND TECHNIQUES

Robert J. McKenna, Jr.

Introduction

The principles of video-assisted thoracic surgery (VATS) are described in this chapter. Although thoracic surgeons may use many techniques to perform minimally invasive operations, my techniques are highlighted in the following paragraphs.

Key Points

- Minimally invasive surgery is good for patients.
- Surgeons can use VATS for most standard operations that previously required a thoracotomy.
- Standard instruments and simple techniques can ensure these procedures are safe for patients.

Definition and Philosophy

A VATS procedure is not a compromise operation; it is the same operation that can be performed by a thoracotomy.[1,2] The standard operation is performed with visualization on a monitor and through incisions without spreading the ribs. Procedures such as a video-assisted lobectomy provide the same complete cancer operation that is performed through a thoracotomy.[3–12]

Indications for an operation usually do not change because the procedure can be performed with minimally invasive surgery. VATS can be performed with standard instruments that are used for open procedures. Articulating instruments are not required. Proper placement of the incisions is essential for successful completion of an operation by VATS techniques.

Positioning

- The position of the patient, monitors, and lights should be set before preparing the patient.
- For most VATS procedures, the patient is placed in the lateral decubitus position with a slight posterior tilt. The patient is taped in place. The arms are at 90 degrees, with the elbows bent in a praying position and with two pillows between the arms. Padding

between the arm board and the downside elbow minimizes the risk of compression causing damage to the ulnar nerve.

- The operating table is flexed with the patient's anterior-superior iliac crest positioned over the flexion of the table. This opens the rib spaces, and this position shifts the hip out of the way so it does not interfere with the movement of the thoracoscope.
- The monitors are placed above the head of the operating table so that the surgeon and all assistants have an unobstructed view of the monitors (Figure 1-1). The surgeon stands on the anterior side of the patient.
- Different positioning may be used for other video-assisted thoracic operations. For example, a Heller myotomy is performed with the monitors at the foot of the bed.

Incisions

Placement of the incisions (Figure 1-2) is key to the performance of VATS. Proper placement of the incisions creates the best angles for the instruments to perform these procedures.

Incision 1

- Incision 1 is 2 cm long and placed in the intercostal space that is just below the infra-mammary crease. It is placed as far anteriorly and inferiorly as possible (approximately the sixth intercostal space in the midclavicular line).
- The incision through the chest wall is angled posteriorly so that it automatically directs instruments through this incision toward the major fissure and away from the pericardium.
- Creation of this incision first allows air into the pleural space so the lung can decompress.
- A finger through this incision confirms that there is no pleural symphysis. If one is detected, blunt dissection is performed to create a space for the trocar to pass through incision 2.
- A finger through this incision protects the diaphragm and liver as the trocar is placed through incision 2.

Incision 2

- Incision 2 is used for the trocar and thoracoscope.
- It is placed low in the chest to provide a panoramic view of the chest. It is in the eighth intercostal space in the posterior axillary line.
- It is angled superiorly so that there is less torque on the intercostal nerve.

Incision 3

- Incision 3 is a utility incision through which much of the dissection is performed and through which a lobe is removed.
- It extends 4 to 6 cm anteriorly from the border of the latissimus dorsi muscle.
- The location of the interspace for the incision is based on the superior pulmonary vein. Through incision 1, a ring forceps pushes the lung posteriorly to expose the superior pulmonary vein. Pressure on the chest wall helps to identify the interspace that is directly up from the vein. That space is used for an upper lobectomy, and one space lower is used for a middle or lower lobectomy.
- Digital palpation of almost all areas of the lung is possible through this incision. I have been able to palpate 3-mm masses through this incision.

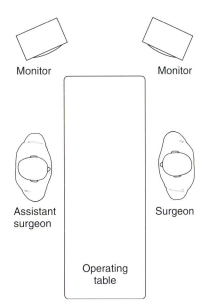

Figure 1-1. Setup for VATS. The monitors are placed above the head of the bed, and the surgeon stands anteriorly.

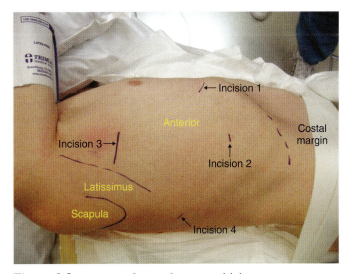

Figure 1-2. Incisions for a video-assisted lobectomy.

Incision 4

- Incision 4 is 1 cm long and placed in the space in the auscultatory triangle.
- It is approximately 3 fingerbreadths below the tip of the scapula and halfway to the spine.
- A slightly higher incision provides slightly better access to help with the paratracheal node dissection. A slightly lower incision provides a better angle for the stapler to cross the superior pulmonary vein.

Instruments

- Standard thoracotomy instruments are the mainstay for VATS. Although there are instruments for thoracoscopic procedures, open instruments are primarily used.
- We primarily use 14-inch Metzenbaum scissors, 14-inch DeBakey pickups, and curved ring forceps (Figure 1-3).

Visualization and Lenses

- A 5-mm thoracoscope is preferred over a 10-mm thoracoscope because it causes less torque on the intercostal nerves (reducing pain), and video equipment can provide excellent visualization through small thoracoscopes.
- A 30-degree lens allows the surgeon to see around structures better than a 0-degree lens.
- A more panoramic view of the pleural space usually is preferable to a closer view. The wider view provides a better understanding of the overall anatomy. When using electrocautery, a wider view shows nearby structures such as nerves and blood vessels, which may be inadvertently cut if not directly visualized. I often tell our residents that if their instinct is to move closer with the camera, they should instead back up the camera.
- A rigid/flexible endoscope (Olympus, Center Valley, Penn) can be helpful, but it requires an experienced person to control it.

Operative Techniques and Complications

Decompression of the Lung

- A double-lumen tube is preferable to a bronchial blocker for VATS because the larger channel of the double-lumen tube enables better lung decompression.
- Clamp the double-lumen tube early (as soon as the patient is positioned for preparation or before turning) to begin the lung decompression.
- Fiberoptic bronchoscopy is important.
  - ▲ To confirm proper placement of the tube after intubation
  - ▲ For suctioning in the mainstem bronchus to decompress the lung (better than a suction catheter)
  - ▲ To evaluate the position of the tube if the patient desaturates during the procedure, or if the decompressed lung begins to expand, or to be ventilated during the procedure
- Right-sided double-lumen tubes is preferred for left-sided operations and left-sided tubes for right-sided operations because a contralateral tube is needed for a sleeve resection, because it is easier for a pneumonectomy (compared with manipulation of an ipsilateral tube during a pneumonectomy), and because the anesthesiologist is comfortable with right-sided tubes when they are really needed, as for a left pneumonectomy or a left sleeve resection.

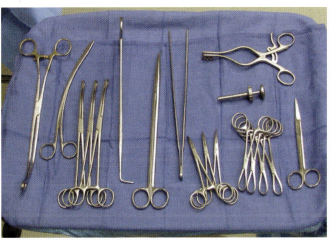

Figure 1-3. Standard instruments used for a video-assisted lobectomy.

Hypoxia During Video-Assisted Thoracic Surgery

- Hypoxia usually is related to improper positioning of the tube.
- Bronchoscopy should be performed to determine if a left-sided tube is too low in the bronchus, causing only the left lower lobe to be ventilated, or to see if a right-sided tube is out of position and the Murphy hole is not aligned correctly with the right upper lobe bronchus.
- Occasionally, the surgeon needs to break scrub to check the positioning of the tube.
- Patients almost never require continuous positive airway pressure (CPAP) or temporary ventilation of the operated lung.

Dissection

- Dissect on named structures (e.g., pulmonary artery, pericardium). Dissecting in the fat may seem safer to a novice, but the anatomy is clearer when named structures are clearly visualized, and the major vessels and nerves are better seen and better protected.
- Surgeons can use sharp or blunt dissection. Simply pushing on a pulmonary artery with the Metzenbaum scissors often defines the vessel.
- Through the utility incision, DeBakey pickups can lift the soft tissue, and Metzenbaum scissors can dissect around vessels (Figure 1-4), or blunt dissection may be performed with the tip of the Yankauer suction or a peanut.
- Pulmonary vessels can be safely lifted with instruments. This maneuver better defines the deeper margin of the vessel. A good purchase on the vessel makes lifting the vessel safer, but a tiny purchase on a vessel increases the likelihood of tearing the vessel.

Stapling Blood Vessels

- Spreading the right angle widely behind the vessel creates a tunnel for the stapler to transect the vessel (Figure 1-5). The stapler requires a large tunnel.
- The anvil passes behind the vessel into the tunnel that has been created by spreading the right angle. Surgeons primarily use endoscopic staples (EZ 45, Ethicon EndoSurgery, Cincinnati, Ohio; Endo-GIA, Covidien, Mansfield, Mass).
- Articulating staples are not needed if the incisions are placed properly.
- There are several methods to safely pass a stapler across a vessel.
  - ▲ Usually, passing the stapler from the proper angle allows the anvil of the stapler to pass through the tunnel behind the vessel.
  - ▲ Occasionally, a tie placed around the vessel lifts it to facilitate passing the stapler across the vessel (Figure 1-6A and B).
  - ▲ Alternatively, pass an 8-mm, red Robinson-Nelaton (Rob-Nel) catheter around the vessel. The anvil of the stapler is placed into the wide end of the Rob-Nel catheter. Leading the Rob-Nel catheter positions the stapler across the vessel (Figure 1-6C and D).
- Be prepared for the possibility of bleeding from a staple line. The thoracoscope should be retracted so vision is not compromised if there is bleeding, the scrub nurse should have a sponge stick available, and the surgeon should have a ring forceps in the incision to apply pressure as needed.

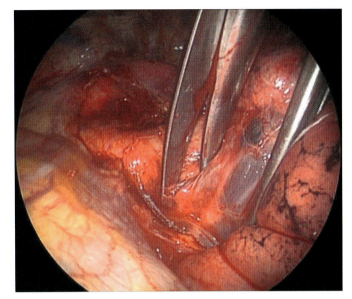

Figure 1-4. Dissection around pulmonary vein.

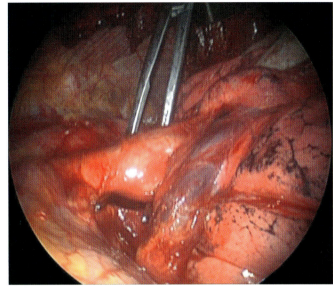

Figure 1-5. Spreading a right angle creates a tunnel for stapling.

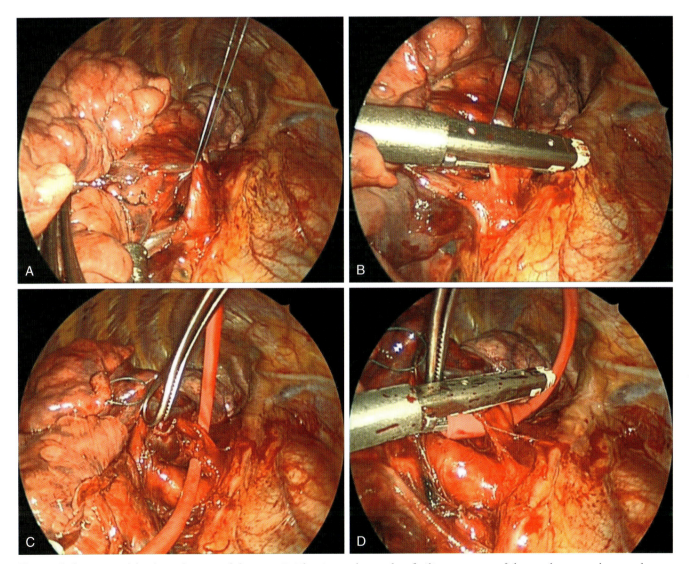

Figure 1-6. A, A tie lifts the right upper lobe vein. **B,** The tie can be used to facilitate passage of the stapler around a vessel. **C,** Alternatively, a red Rob-Nel catheter can be placed around the vessel. **D,** This catheter can be used to pass the stapler around the vessel.

Alternative Techniques for Vessels

- Staples may be too large and may be an unnecessary expense for smaller vessels.
- Small vessels can be clipped with standard clips used during thoracotomy (Figure 1-7).
- Vessels may be tied with standard extracorporeal knot tying. Through the utility incision, a finger can pass the tie to the vessel (Figure 1-8). Knot pushers are also available (Figure 1-9).
- A suture ligature may be used.

Stapling Parenchyma

- Surgeons primarily use endoscopic staples (EZ 45, Endo-GIA) to complete a fissure or perform a nonanatomic wedge resection.
- Articulating staples are not needed if the incisions are placed properly. The mobile lung can be positioned properly into the jaw of the stapler.
- Pass the stapler carefully across the lung parenchyma so that the device is parallel to the surfaces of the lung, rather than poking into the lung parenchyma (Figure 1-10).
- When completing the fissure, place the anvil of the stapler on the pulmonary artery. Hold the stapler in that position as the parenchyma is pulled into the device. This protects the pulmonary vessels and minimizes the chances of damage to the vessels or inadvertent transaction of a vessel.

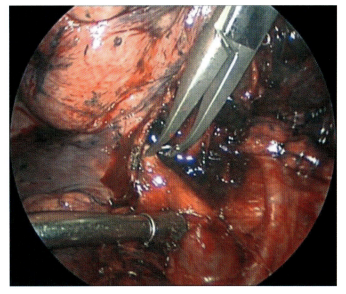

Figure 1-7. Placement of a clip for a small pulmonary artery.

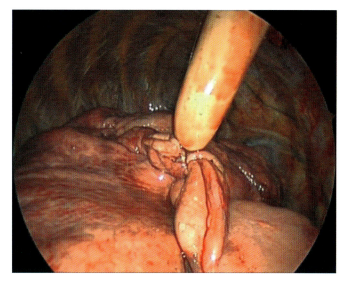

Figure 1-8. Tying a small vessel.

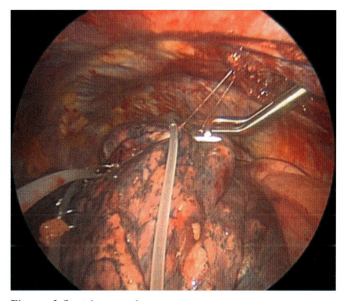

Figure 1-9. A knot pusher.

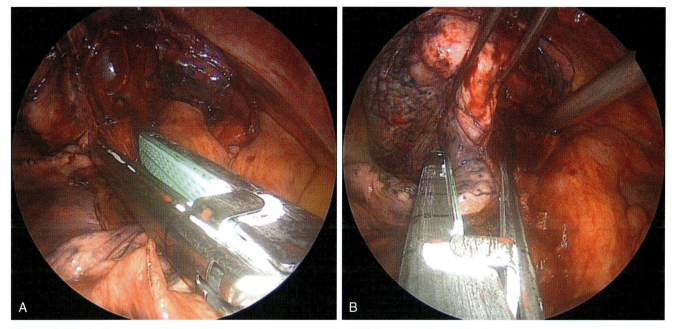

Figure 1-10. A, Correct positioning for the stapler to transect the RUL bronchus **B,** and the fissure.

Suturing

- The ability to suture is important for advanced VATS procedures.
- Endoscopic needle holders are unnecessary. A standard needle holder or a thoracoscopic needle driver can be inserted through the utility incision. The mobile lung can be moved so that the tissue is aligned for suturing (Figure 1-11).
- Knots are tied outside the body in the same fashion as for a thoracotomy. A finger can push the knots to the tissue. If the tissue is too far away, a ring forceps can bring it closer to the incision. Rarely is a knot pusher needed.

Removal of Specimens

- All specimens that may be cancer should be removed in a bag to minimize the chance of tumor recurrence in an incision.
- Smaller specimens can be removed in a tissue bag (EndoCatch, Covidien).
- Larger specimens, such as a lobe, are placed in a larger bag for removal (LapSac, Cook, Bloomington, Indiana) (Figure 1-12). Removing an entire lobe through a 4- to 6-cm incision requires a strong pull, and smaller bags break with a strong pull.

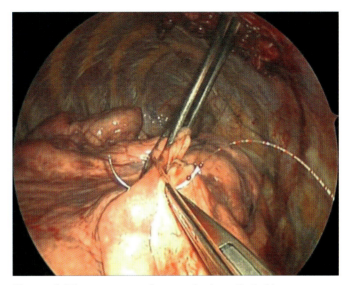

Figure 1-11. Suturing with a standard needle holder.

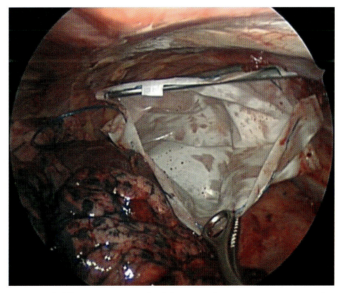

Figure 1-12. Placement of a lobe into the LapSac tissue pouch.

References

1. McKenna RJ Jr, Houck W, Fuller CB: Video-assisted thoracic surgery lobectomy: experience with 1100 cases, *Ann Thorac Surg* 81:421–426, 2006.
2. Onaitis MW, Petersen RP, Balderson SS, et al: Thoracoscopic lobectomy is a safe and versatile procedure: experience with 500 consecutive patients, *Ann Surg* 244:420–425, 2006.
3. Mahtabifard A, Fuller CB, McKenna RJ Jr: VATS sleeve lobectomy, *Ann Thorac Surg* 85(2):5279–5332, 2008.
4. McKenna RJ Jr, Mahtabifard A, Fuller CB: Fast tracking after VATS pulmonary resection, *Ann Thorac Surg* 84(5):1663–1667, 2007.
5. Cerfolio RJ, Bass C, Katholi CR: Prospective, randomized trial compares suction versus water seal for air leaks, *Ann Thorac Surg* 73:1727–1731, 2002.
6. Whitson BA, Boettcher A, Bardales R, Kratzke RA, Dahlberg PS, Andrade RS, Maddaus MA: Comparison of video assisted thoracoscopic surgery to thoracotomy for resection of clinical stage I non-small cell lung cancer. Presented at the American College of Surgeons Congress, Chicago, IL, October 10, 2006.
7. Nomori H, Ohtsuka T, Horio H, et al: Difference in the impairment of vital capacity and 6-minute walking after a lobectomy performed by thoracoscopic surgery, an anterior limited thoracotomy, an antero-axillary thoracotomy, and a posterolateral thoracotomy, *Surg Today* 33:7–12, 2003.
8. Nakata M, Saeki H, Yokoyama N, et al: Pulmonary function after lobectomy: video-assisted thoracic surgery versus thoracotomy, *Ann Thorac Surg* 70:938–941, 2000.
9. Demmy TL, Curtis JJ: Minimally invasive lobectomy directed toward frail and high-risk patients: a case-control study, *Ann Thorac Surg* 68:194–200, 1999.
10. Demmy TL, Plante AJ, Nwogu CE, et al: Discharge independence with minimally invasive lobectomy, *Am J Surg* 188:698–702, 2004.
11. Nakajima J, Takamoto S, Kohno T, Ohtsuka T: Costs of videothoracoscopic surgery versus open resection for patients with lung carcinoma, *Cancer* 89(Suppl):2497–2501, 2000.
12. Petersen RP, Pham D, Burfeind WR, et al: Thoracoscopic lobectomy facilitates the delivery of chemotherapy after resection for lung cancer, *Ann Thorac Surg* 83:1245–1249; discussion 1250, 2007.

CHAPTER 2

VIDEO–ASSISTED THORACIC SURGERY VERSUS THORACOTOMY: IMPACT ON THE IMMUNE SYSTEM

Robert J. McKenna, III

Introduction

Minimally invasive surgery is attractive to patients for many reasons, such as smaller scars, shorter hospital stays, and earlier recovery. Although the lower complication rates after minimally invasive surgery usually have been attributed to patients experiencing less pain, the lower complication rates may reflect a more intact immune system after minimally invasive surgery.[1]

Surgery causes immunosuppression by "hemodynamic changes in humoral agents, such as catecholamines, and by peptides, such as cytokines, produced at the site of injury and by various immune cells."[2] Immunosuppression can increase the likelihood of tumor metastasis formation and development of septic complications postoperatively.[3] Lord Moynihan of Leeds said, "The cleaner and gentler the act of operation, the less the patient suffers, the smoother and quicker his convalescence, the more exquisite the wound heals."[4]

Some surgeons theorize that minimally invasive surgery may increase cancer cure rates by reducing the impact of an operation on the immune system. This chapter explores that theory and compares the data on minimally invasive thoracic surgery (i.e., video-assisted thoracic surgery [VATS]) and on open thoracotomy for lung cancer surgery:

- In a randomized, prospective study for lobectomy, VATS had a significantly lower complication rate than thoracotomy (14.2% versus 50%, $P = .03$).[5]
- The National Emphysema Treatment Trial showed earlier recovery and fewer health care costs after VATS compared with a median sternotomy for lung volume reduction surgery.[6]
- Many other comparisons of VATS and historic controls have been published.[1,5,7,10]
- VATS has been associated with a reduced impact on measurable components of the immune system[1,7,8] and possibly with higher cure rates for lung cancer surgery,[9,10] leading to speculation about whether patient selection or the procedure's diminished immunologic disturbance may account for improved outcomes.

Surgery, Cancer, and the Immune System

Human studies have shown that patients with compromised immune systems are at increased risk for developing cancer.[11] In a prospective study over 11 years, the age-adjusted cancer risk was 0.63 for subjects with normal cytotoxic activity compared with patients with compromised cytotoxic activity.[11]

It is thought that a normally functioning human immune system regularly scavenges and removes aberrant cells.[12] For example, despite the fact that cancer cells are found in the blood of patients after lung cancer surgery,[13] many are cured by the operations, indicating that the immune system must control the circulating cancer cells.

The balance between the cancer burden and immune system status may affect the body's ability to control the cancer. Surgical stress may lessen immunologic activity, and the type of procedure may affect tumor cell dissemination. For example, in a comparison of female C3H/He mice treated by laparotomy or laparoscopy, tumor nodules subsequently developed in 5%, 30%, and 83% (P <.01) of the control mice, laparoscopic resection mice, and open resection mice, respectively.[14]

Surgical Stress and Immunologic Function

In general, surgery has been shown to compromise the immune system.[7] Surgery induces the release of acute-phase response mediators, such as C-reactive protein (CRP) and cytokines, whose concentration increases or decreases in response to inflammation.[1] In an acute inflammatory and immunologic response to injury or trauma, neutrophil granulocytes and macrophages secrete molecules known as cytokines into the bloodstream. Important cytokines include interleukins IL-1, IL-6, and IL-8 and tumor necrosis factor (TNF).

The liver responds by producing a large number of acute-phase reactants, such as CRP, which inhibits the growth of microbes by binding to phosphorylcholine, assists in complement binding to foreign and damaged cells, and enhances phagocytosis by macrophages. CRP may increase 50,000-fold in response to acute inflammation and infection, initially. Because this occurs within 6 hours and peaks at 48 hours, measuring and charting CRP values can help to determine disease progress or the effectiveness of treatments.[15]

TNF, primarily produced by macrophages, can promote apoptotic cell death, cellular proliferation, differentiation, inflammation, tumorigenesis, and viral replication. TNF causes the hypothalamus to suppress appetite and induce fever. TNF causes the liver to stimulate an acute-phase response that increases CRP and other mediators and it attracts neutrophils to help them stick to endothelial cells for migration. TNF causes macrophages to stimulate phagocytosis and the production of IL-1 oxidants and inflammatory lipid prostaglandin E_2 (PGE_2). A locally increased concentration causes inflammation, including heat, swelling, redness, and pain. Overproduction and high concentrations of TNF may induce shocklike symptoms, and it has been implicated in a variety of human diseases, including cancer.[16] Several laparoscopic procedures have provoked a smaller release of cytokines than open laparotomies.[1,17]

Immune effector cells (IECs) are short-lived, activated cells that defend the body in an immune response. Effector B and T cells, also known as plasma cells, secrete antibodies and cytotoxic (CD8) and helper (CD4) cells that carry out cell-mediated responses. Some IECs are less affected by minimally invasive surgery than open procedures. With compromised IECs, established tumors grew equally well after minimally invasive surgery and open surgery,[14] but with intact IECs, tumor growth rate was significantly greater after an open procedure.[18] In a male Wrister rat (350 to 380 g) model, the effects of stress (i.e., corticosteroid) and immunologic parameters (i.e., neopterin and IL-1β).[18] were compared for laparoscopic and open surgery.

Anabolic parameters reflect the immunologic effect of surgical stress. Significant differences were found in postoperative stress (491 versus 609 ng/mL, P = .08) and immune parameters (neopterin: 0.225 versus 0.372 ng/mL, P = .01; IL-1β: 268 versus 754 pg/mL, P = .2). Seven days postoperatively, the rats lost 5.99% of their body weight after open surgery and only 2.4% after laparoscopic surgery. Weight loss is a reflection of the anabolic state of the rats.[19]

Insulin-like growth factor 1 (IGF-1) is another parameter of anabolism that may play an important role in malignant cell propagation; postoperative decreases in serum levels of IGF correlate with the degree of surgical trauma. Assisting in metabolism, growth, and regeneration, IGF-1 travels to extracellular tissue. In male rats of the inbred WAG strain

(200 to 300 g), Bouvy and colleagues[20] found significantly higher total peritoneal tumor load for conventional open small-bowel resection ($P < .05$) compared with higher postoperative IGF-1 levels for laparoscopic procedures ($P < .02$). However, these findings are not specific because there are other factors that influence the immune system and tumor growth. Operations may cause localized ischemia that reduces defense mechanisms, which makes the ischemic site vulnerable for tumor implantation and growth.[20] This is a complex issue because even the type of insufflation used for laparoscopic procedures affects tumor growth. Because of a greater effect on hemodynamics, carbon dioxide (compared with helium) insufflation promotes tumor growth.[21]

There are much more data for abdominal operations than for thoracic operations. However, comparisons of the immune response to VATS with that for open thoracotomy suggest that minimally invasive procedures in the chest may also have immunologic benefits.[7,8]

The immune system response to surgical trauma is a complex interaction of several systems. Changes in the immune system may affect the immediate postoperative period. Cytokines trigger or enhance endothelial leukocyte activation.[1,7,8] Although elevated IL-6 levels correlate with the degree of surgical trauma, they are more than a marker of the degree of trauma. Cytokines are the main mediators of the inflammatory response. IL-6 is the main inducer of liver synthesis of acute-phase proteins.[22] IL-6 is also involved in rapid weight loss, which frequently accompanies short-term disease or injury such as sepsis, trauma, or burns.[22] Hypermetabolism-associated malnutrition in liver transplant recipients is involved in the deterioration of perioperative energy metabolism and the exaggerated postoperative IL-6 response. IL-6 is an important mediator of experimental cancer cachexia in the murine adenocarcinoma cell line.[7] Some human studies have shown an increased IL-6 response in nutritionally depleted cancer patients.[23]

Increased levels of certain proinflammatory cytokines, such as IL-6 and IL-8, caused by surgical trauma increase the risk of postoperative complications.[1] Recruited by inflammation, primary macrophage cells process antigens and release chemokines to signal other cells. One such chemokine, IL-8, induces chemotaxis in its target cells, such as neutrophil granulocytes, to phagocytose the antigen, which triggers pattern toll-like receptors. Some studies comparing laparoscopy with open laparotomy for colectomy,[24] hysterectomy,[25] and Nissen fundoplication[26] show that the minimally invasive procedure causes less release of CRP, whereas other studies did not show that laparoscopy had less impact on the immune system.[27]

Thoracic Surgery and the Immune System

In a prospective comparison of lobectomy patients undergoing VATS or thoracotomy for lung cancer, the postoperative levels of IL-6 and IL-8 were significantly lower in the VATS group.[28] Previously, Yamada and colleagues showed that high IL-6 and IL-8 levels after thoracic surgical procedures were associated with an increased incidence of postoperative infections[28] and respiratory failure.[29,30] Szczesny and coworkers showed that elevated levels of IL-6 in pleural fluid was a marker for a higher risk of postoperative complications.[31]

The data about thoracic procedures and the immune system are not clear-cut. Sugi and coworkers[32] found no difference in the IL-6 and IL-8 levels for VATS and thoracotomy patients,[1] and Friscia and associates[33] showed lower levels of IL-6 and IL-8 for VATS compared with open lung volume reduction surgery.

Cancer Development and the Immune System

Changes in the immune system may affect the body's ability to fight cancer. Elevated IL-6 levels may encourage cell proliferation in certain subtypes of non–small-cell lung cancer.[34] Because it promotes the activity of insulin growth factor (IGF) and inhibits IGF binding protein (IGFBP), IL-6 creates an environment that may promote tumor growth.[32] IGF may cause progression of tumors because it stimulates tumor growth and reduces tumor apoptosis.[35] Because IGFBP attenuates the activity of IGF, it inhibits tumorigenesis. Low circulating levels of IGFBP have been found in patients with advanced prostate cancer[36] and patients at risk for colon cancer.[32] The anti-oncogenic properties of IGFBP-3 include the induction of apoptosis in lung cancer[37] and impairment of DNA synthesis in poorly differentiated tumor cells.[32] IL-12, IL-17, and IL-23 are less affected by VATS than open procedures, but the significance of this is unknown.[7]

IGFBP-3 may be particularly important in lung cancer patients. Patients after lung cancer surgery have circulating cancer cells.[13] In a prospective study, IGFBP-3 levels were higher on postoperative day 3 for patients after VATS than after thoracotomy. Conversely, levels of matrix metalloproteinase 9 (MMP-9), which cleaves and deactivates IGFBP-3, were lower in the VATS patients. Elevated MMP-9 levels facilitate tumor invasion and metastasis through its proteolytic properties against type IV collagen in the basement membrane.[38,39] These data suggest that there may be an immunologic reason why VATS may provide better lung cancer survival than a thoracotomy.

Surgery and Cellular Immunity

Most operations diminish circulating lymphocytes and cell-mediated immunity, and minimally invasive procedures appear to have a smaller impact on the immune system. For abdominal surgery, laparoscopy has a smaller impact than a laparotomy.[7]

VATS produces less immunosuppression of lymphocytes and causes a smaller reduction in the total number of T cells and CD4 T cells. Natural killer (NK) cells are important for tumor immunosurveillance because they recognize, target, and kill tumor cells without prior sensitization.[40] The number of NK cells is considerably lower after thoracotomy than after VATS.[41] IL-10 is a cytokine that helps tumor cells escape from the immune system by inhibiting NK cell cytotoxicity, and in experiments, it increased tumor cell resistance to NK cells.[42] After lobectomy, IL-10 levels are higher. Phagocytosis by neutrophils is less affected after VATS.[8,32]

Components of the cellular immune system may be affected less after a minimally invasive operation than after an operation through large traditional incisions. Compared with thoracotomy,[1,7,8] VATS is associated with better cellular immunity (i.e., neutrophil and monocyte function) and less postoperative impact on CRP, causes fewer disturbances of chemokines, and produces a lower stress response. The degree of access trauma correlates with the degree of inflammation and immunosuppression. The reduced impact of VATS may translate into better survival for cancer patients who have minimally invasive surgery.

Experiments with a delayed-type hypersensitivity (DTH) assay, which evaluates the cellular immune system, have shown that laparotomy has a greater impact on the cellular immune system than laparoscopy. The DTH response starts with antigen injected into the skin. In the activation phase, antigen is presented to lymphocytes on the surface of antigen-presenting cells. In the inflammatory phase, antigen-stimulated CD4$^+$ lymphocytes respond by proliferating and elaborating cytokines that act in an endocrine manner to cause endothelial cell leakage and fibrin deposition that creates swelling at the site of antigen challenge. In the effector phase, vascular endothelial cells, activated by cytokines, recruit effector cells to eliminate the intracellular pathogen. The size of the induration of the skin is directly proportional to the strength of the immune response. Anergy to DTH testing is associated with a significantly higher incidence of postoperative sepsis, wound infection, mortality, and even lower resectability rates and higher cancer recurrence rates.[43]

DTH testing has been used to assess the impact of open compared with minimally invasive abdominal surgery in animals. Gleason and colleagues[43] studied three serial DTH challenges of phytohemagglutinin (PHA) in 100 5- to 6-week-old female C3H/H3N mice. PHA is a polyclonal stimulator that acts directly on immature CD4$^+$ lymphocytes, stimulating cell proliferation and cytokine production. Measurements of footpad thickness showed a significantly lower DTH response in the sham laparotomy group compared with the laparoscopy group, indicating cellular immune suppression in the open group.[43]

Suppression of the cellular immune system increases susceptibility to sepsis. In two similar rat models testing cell-mediated immune function, Allendorf and colleagues[44] compared laparotomy with pneumoperitoneum, and in another study, Allendorf and coworkers[45] compared laparoscopy with laparotomy. They tested the susceptibility to bacterial infections by measuring the size of skin pustules after injection with *Staphylococcus aureus* 502A. Both groups showed better cellular immune function with the minimally invasive surgery, as demonstrated by smaller pustules and quicker healing. When researchers gauged immune function by evaluating DTH responses to phytohemagglutinin (PHA), a nonspecific T-cell mitogen, he found significantly smaller DTH response in the laparotomy group.[18]

Conclusions

Compared with thoracotomy, VATS may have a reduced impact on the immune system that may lead to fewer healing or infectious problems in the short term and better survival in the long run. VATS leads to better preservation of cellular immunity. It compromises inflammatory and immunomodulatory mediators less and impacts tumor biology less than thoracotomy.

Open surgery reduces lymphocyte and neutrophil chemotaxis, NK cell activity, lymphocyte and macrophage interactions, and DTH responses. Diminished immunologic function increases the likelihood of sepsis and tumor metastasis.

The data are more extensive and stronger for abdominal surgery, but the data regarding thoracic surgery are increasing. Mounting evidence suggests that there are good reasons to offer more patients minimally invasive thoracic surgery.

References

1. Yim AP, Wan S, Lee TW, Arifi AA: VATS lobectomy reduces cytokine responses compared with conventional surgery, *Ann Thorac Surg* 70:243–247, 2000.
2. Vallina VL, Velasco JM: The influence of laparoscopy on lymphocyte subpopulations in the surgical patient, *Surg Endosc* 10:481–484, 1996.
3. Lennard TW, Shenton BK, Borzotta A, et al: The influence of surgical operation on the components of the immune system, *Br J Surg* 72:771–776, 1985.
4. Buckman RF: Lord Moynihan of Leeds, *Surg Gynecol Obstet* 142:90–94, 1976.
5. Hoksch B, Ablassmaier B, Walter M, Muller JM: Complication rate after thoracoscopic and conventional lobectomy, *Zentralbl Chir* 128:106–110, 2003.
6. National Emphysema Treatment Trial (NETT) Research Group: National Emphysema Treatment Trial: a comparison of median sternotomy versus VATS for lung volume reduction surgery, *J Thorac Cardiovasc Surg* 127:1350–1360, 2004.
7. Ng CS, Wan S, Hui CW, et al: Video-assisted thoracic surgery for early stage lung cancer–can short-term immunological advantages improve long-term outcomes? *Ann Thorac Cardiovasc Surg* 12:308–312, 2006.
8. Craig Sr, Leaver HA, Yap PL, Walker WS: Acute phase responses following minimally invasive access and conventional thoracic surgery, *Eur J Cardiothorac Surg* 20:455–639, 2001.
9. Sugi K, Sudoh M, Hirazawa K, et al: Intrathoracic bleeding during video-assisted thoracoscopic lobectomy and segmentectomy, *Kyobu Geka* 56:928–931, 2003.
10. Kaseda S, Aoki T: Video-assisted thoracic surgical lobectomy in conjunction with lymphadenectomy for lung cancer, *Nippon Geka Gakkai Zasshi* 103:717–721, 2002.
11. Imai K, Matsuyama S, Miyake S, et al: Natural cytotoxic activity of peripheral-blood lymphocytes and cancer incidence: an 11 year follow up study of a general population, *Lancet* 356:1795–1799, 2000.
12. Whitsen BA, D'Cunha J, Maddaus MA: Minimally invasive surgery improves patients' survival rates through less perioperative immunosuppression, *Med Hypotheses* 68:1328–1332, 2007.
13. Yamashita JI, Kurusu Y, Fujino N, et al: Detection of circulating tumor cells in patients with non-small cell lung cancer undergoing lobectomy by video-assisted thoracic surgery: a potential hazard for intraoperative hematogenous tumor cell dissemination, *J Thorac Cardiovasc Surg* 119:899–905, 2000.
14. Allendorf JD, Bessler M, Horvath KD, et al: Increased tumor establishment and growth after open vs laparoscopic surgery may be related to differences in postoperative lymphocyte function, *Surg Endosc* 13:233–235, 1997.
15. Pepys MB, Hirshfield GM: C-reactive protein: a critical update, *J Clin Invest* 111:1805–1812, 2003.
16. Locksley RM, Killeen N, Lenardo MJ: The TNF and TNF receptor superfamilies: integrating mammalian biology, *Cell* 104:487–501, 2001.
17. Vittimberga FJ, Foley DP, Meyers WC, Callery MP: Laparoscopic surgery and the immune response, *Ann Surg* 227:326–334, 1998.
18. Allendorf JD, Bessler M, Whelan RL, et al: Postoperative immune function varies inversely with the degree of surgical trauma in murine model, *Surg Endosc* 11:427–430, 1997.
19. Kuntz C, Wunch A, Bay F, et al: Prospective randomized study of stress and immune response after laparoscopic vs conventional colonic resection, *Surg Endosc* 12:963–967, 1998.
20. Bouvy ND, Marquet RL, Jeekel J, Bonjer HJ: Laparoscopic surgery is associated with less tumor growth stimulation than conventional surgery: an experimental study, *Br J Surg* 84:358–361, 1997.
21. Gut CN, Kuntz C, Schmandra TH, et al: *Metabolism and immunology in laparoscopy. First workshop on experimental laparoscopic surgery, Surg Endo* 12(8):1096–1098, 1997.
22. Wan S, LeClerc JL, Vincent JL: Cytokine responses to cardiopulmonary bypass: lessons learned from cardiac transplantation, *Ann Thorac Surg* 63:269–276, 1997.
23. Nakagoe T, Tsuji T, Sawai T, et al: Increased serum levels of interleukin-6 in malnourished patients with colorectal cancer, *Cancer Lett* 202:109–115, 2003.

24. Harmon GD, Senagone AJ, Kilbride MJ, Warzynski MJ: Interleukin response to laparoscopic and open cholecystectomy, *Dis Colon Rectum* 37:754–759, 1994.
25. Ellstrom M, Bengtsson A, Tylman M, et al: Evaluation of tissue trauma after laparoscopic and abdominal hysterectomy: measurements of neutrophil activation and release of interleukin-6, cortisol, and C-reactive protein, *J Am Coll Surg* 182:423–430, 1996.
26. Siestes C, Wiezer MJ, Eijsbouts QA, et al: A prospective, randomized study of the systemic immune response after laparoscopic and conventional Nissen fundoplication, *Surgery* 126:5–9, 1999.
27. Brune IB, Wilke W, Hensler T, et al: Downregulation of T helper type 1 immune response and altered pro-inflammatory and anti-inflammatory T cell cytokine balance following conventional but not laparoscopic surgery, *Am J Surg* 177:55–60, 1999.
28. Yamada T, Hisanaga M, Nakajima Y, et al: Serum interleukin-6, interleukin-8, hepatocyte growth factor, and nitric oxide changes during thoracic surgery, *World J Surg* 22:783–790, 1998.
29. Katsuta T, Saito T, Shigemitsu Y, et al: Relation between tumor necrosis factor alpha and interleukin 1 beta producing capacity of peripheral monocytes and pulmonary complications following oesophagectomy, *Br J Surg* 85:548–553, 1998.
30. Takeda S, Takeda S, Kim C, et al: Preoperative administration of methylprednisolone attenuates cytokine-induced respiratory failure after esophageal resection, *J Nippon Med Sch* 70:16–20, 2003.
31. Szczesny TJ, Slotwinski R, Stankiewicz A, et al: Interleukin-6 and interleukin 1 receptor antagonist as early markers of postoperative complications after lung cancer surgery, *Eur J Cardiothorac Surg* 31:719–724, 2007.
32. Sugi K, Kaneda Y, Esato K: Video-assisted thoracoscopic lobectomy reduces cytokine production more than conventional open lobectomy, *J Thorac Cardiovasc Surg* 48:161–165, 2000.
33. Friscia ME, Jianliang Z, Kolff JW, et al: Cytokine response is lower after lung volume reduction surgery through bilateral thoracoscopy versus sternotomy, *Ann Thorac Surg* 83:252–256, 2007.
34. Chang KT, Tsai CM, Chiou YC, et al: IL-6 induces neuroendocrine dedifferentiation and cell proliferation in non-small cell lung cancer cells, *Am J Physiol Lung Cell Mol Physiol* 289:L447–L453, 2005.
35. Wu Y, Yakar S, Zhao L, et al: Circulating insulin-like growth factor-1 levels regulate colon cancer growth and metastases, *Cancer Res* 62:10301–10335, 2002.
36. Shariat SF, Lamb DJ, Kattan MW, et al: Association of preoperative plasma levels of insulin-like levels of growth factor binding proteins-2 and -3 with prostate cancer invasion, progression, and metastasis, *J Clin Oncol* 20:833–841, 2002.
37. Chang YS, Kong G, Sun S, et al: Clinical significance of insulin-like growth factor-binding protein-3 expression in stage 1 nonsmall cell lung cancer, *Clin Cancer Res* 8:3796–3802, 2002.
38. Liotta LA, Tryggvason K, Garbisa S, et al: Metastatic potential correlates enzymatic degradation of basement membrane collagen, *Nature* 284:67–68, 1980.
39. Iizasa T, Fujisawa T, Suzuki M, et al: Elevated levels of circulating plasma matrix metalloproteinase 9 in non-small cell lung cancer patients, *Clin Cancer Res* 5:149–153, 1999.
40. Ng CS, Lee TW, Wan S, et al: Thoracotomy is associated with significantly more profound suppression in lymphocytes and natural killer cells than video assisted thoracic surgery following major lung resection for cancer, *J Invest Surg* 18:81–88, 2005.
41. Leaver HA, Craig SR, Yap PL, Walker WS: Lymphocyte responses following open and minimally invasive thoracic surgery, *Eur J Clin Invest* 30:230–238, 2000.
42. Tsuruma T, Yagihashi A, Torigoe T, et al: Interleukin-10 reduces natural killer sensitivity and downregulates MHC class I expression on H-ras-transformed cells, *Cell Immunol* 184:121–128, 1998.
43. Gleason NR, Blanco I, Allendorf JD, et al: Delayed-type hypersensitivity response is better preserved in mice following insufflations than after laparotomy, *Surg Endosc* 13:1032–1034, 1999.
44. Allendorf JDF, Bessler M, Whelan RL, et al: Better preservation of the immune fucntion after laparoscopic-assisted versus open bowl resection in a murine model, *Dis Colon Rectum* 39(Suppl):S67–S72, 1996.
45. Allendorf JDF, Bessler M, Horvath KD, et al: Increased tumor establishment and growth after open vs laproscopic bowl resection in mice, *Surg Endosc* 12:1035–1038, 1998.

CHAPTER 3

ANESTHETIC CONSIDERATIONS

Karen S. Sibert and Robert A. Frantz

Introduction

Anesthesia for minimally invasive thoracic surgery involves many of the same techniques that anesthesiologists use for open thoracic procedures. Successful anesthetic management includes several components:

- Facility with placement and adjustment of right- and left-sided double-lumen endotracheal tubes (DLTs)
- Knowledge of tracheobronchial anatomy and skill with fiberoptic bronchoscopy
- Expertise with thoracic epidural analgesia
- Anesthesiologists dedicated to providing anesthesia for thoracic cases

Patient Preparation and Monitoring

- Most patients are moderate to high anesthesia risks (i.e., American Society of Anesthesiologists [ASA] physical status class 3), and abnormal pulmonary function test results are expected.
- If the patient is on bronchodilator therapy, provide treatment in the preoperative area.
- Discuss postoperative pain management, including the possibility of epidural analgesia.
- Reassuringly prepare the patient to anticipate that breathing will be uncomfortable on waking due to the effect of chest tubes and lung reexpansion.
- Patients who have had neoadjuvant radiation therapy or chemotherapy must be identified in advance and kept on the lowest acceptable F_{IO_2} because they are more susceptible to hyperoxic lung injury.
- A single, reliable, 18-gauge intravenous catheter is adequate for many minimally invasive cases.
- Radial artery catheters are placed for most cases unless the patient is especially healthy or the anticipated procedure is brief.
- Central venous access is required less frequently unless intravenous access is limited or substantial blood loss is anticipated; central lines are routinely placed for pneumonectomy, esophagectomy, and lung volume reduction surgery.

Double-Lumen Endotracheal Tube Placement

Applications
- DLTs are required for most thoracic cases: wedge resection, lobectomy, pneumonectomy, lung reduction, pleurodesis, decortication, and esophagectomy.

◆ They are not required for mediastinoscopy, sympathectomy, or pericardial window (i.e., subxyphoid approach).

◆ We exclusively use DLTs for any procedure requiring lung separation. Bronchial blockers do not allow adequate deflation or suctioning of the operated lung.

◆ Routine use of a video laryngoscope permits full visualization of the DLT tip as it passes between the vocal cords.

Routine Intubation

We developed a 5-step process for passage of the DLT into the larynx, most often with the use of a Mac 4 video laryngoscope.

1. Insert the Mac blade into the right side of the mouth, and use the flange to sweep the tongue over to the left.
2. Advance the tip of the blade into the vallecula, and elevate the blade to reveal the vocal cords. In some patients, the view improves with the tip of the blade beneath the epiglottis.
3. Bend or curve the DLT at an angle of 30 to 45 degrees about 6 to 8 cm from the tip, and insert it from the right side of the mouth so that the tip approaches the vocal cords.
4. Depending on the relationship of the bronchial tip and the surrounding structures, one of two approaches is necessary:
   a. If the alignment is suitable (with or without the stylet in place), pass the DLT beyond the vocal cords into the mid-trachea.
   b. If the tip of the bronchial lumen impinges on the anterior or lateral laryngeal structures (i.e., anterior commissure) or the arytenoid cartilages, gently redirect or rotate the tube to guide the tip past the obstacles. It may be helpful to retract the stylet.
5. Because the DLT is often anteriorly directed at this stage, the leading edge may catch on the tracheal rings, preventing advancement of the tube. Additional gentle rotation and pressure may be necessary to "screw" the DLT into the mid-trachea, and it may be necessary to pass a fiberoptic bronchoscope through the bronchial lumen to help guide the DLT tip through the tracheal rings and into the appropriate bronchus.

Difficult Intubation

◆ Use of a DLT exchange catheter facilitates placement of a DLT in patients with an anterior larynx, limited aperture, or other difficult airway situations (Figure 3-1). The exchange catheter may be guided into the trachea using direct video laryngoscopy or advanced through a previously placed single-lumen endotracheal tube. The DLT is then passed over the catheter into the trachea. Care must be taken to pass the exchange catheter tip gently just past the vocal cords to avoid tracheal injury.

◆ Another safe approach to the difficult airway is to insert a fiberoptic bronchoscope into the trachea and pass the DLT directly over it. Maneuvers including jaw thrust, tongue retraction, and simultaneous laryngoscopy facilitate passage of the tube through the laryngeal inlet.

Achieving Optimal DLT Placement

◆ Correct placement of a DLT can be achieved in one of two accepted ways:
   • Insert the DLT into the trachea, and use fiberoptic bronchoscopy (FOB) to direct the tube down the appropriate mainstem bronchus.
   • Insert the DLT to an estimated appropriate depth in the mainstem bronchus during the initial laryngoscopy (our usual practice), and use FOB to confirm placement and adjust the tube position as necessary.

Choice of Right versus Left DLT

In many institutions, left DLTs are used for all thoracic cases because of the perceived difficulty in situating right-sided tubes properly to ventilate the right upper lobe (RUL). We disagree; we routinely use right DLTs for most left lung cases, and left DLTs for all right lung cases. There are multiple advantages to this approach:

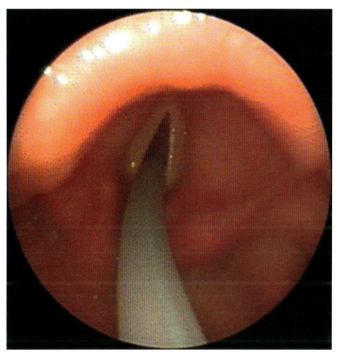

Figure 3-1. Insertion of a soft-tipped exchange catheter into the trachea facilitates passage of a double-lumen endotracheal tube in a patient with a difficult airway.

- There is no risk of inadvertently stapling the cuff of a left DLT during left lobectomy or pneumonectomy.
- A complete view of the carina and the mainstem bronchus of the operated lung is obtained during bronchoscopy.
- Bronchoscopy through the tracheal lumen to check the distal cuff position does not interrupt ventilation of the nonoperated lung.
- If the tracheal (proximal) cuff is damaged by the patient's teeth during insertion, lung isolation is still accomplished by the intact distal cuff.
- If a left DLT is used for left lung surgery, it is possible for pressure on the operated lung to occlude the tracheal lumen, which is ventilating the right lung, or to push the bronchial cuff back into the trachea.
- Right DLTs are easy to insert because the path to the right mainstem bronchus is more direct. A contralateral tube is imperative when a sleeve resection is performed (e.g., if a left-sided tube is used when the left mainstem bronchus is open during a bronchial sleeve), the tube interferes with suturing and the patient is not ventilated well.

Troubleshooting after Initial Insertion

- In 5% to 10% of cases, a left DLT goes down the right mainstem bronchus, despite the usual leftward rotation, as it is advanced. Withdraw the tube into the trachea, and advance it into the left bronchus under direct FOB vision.
- When the patient is turned lateral and flexed, the DLT usually retracts cephalad at least a centimeter and may need to be advanced to avoid herniation of the distal cuff over the carina. This is especially likely in edentulous patients. It is always easier to pull a DLT back than to advance it after it has become warm and flexible.
- Always repeat fiberoptic bronchoscopy after lateral positioning to confirm proper tube placement.
- Hypoxemia is usually a sign of an improperly placed tube; we rarely find it necessary to use continuous positive airway pressure (CPAP) for the operated lung or positive end-expiratory pressure (PEEP) greater than 5 cm to the nonoperated lung. During lobectomy, the oxygen saturation always improves after clamping of the arterial blood supply to the lobe.
- With a right DLT, if the distance to the takeoff of the RUL bronchus is very short, the distal cuff may herniate over the carina. In this event, connect the FOB to suction, and pass it down the left mainstem bronchus to deflate the left lung.
- After the patient is positioned laterally, the alignment of the RUL orifice on a right DLT may be altered. It may be difficult to regain perfect alignment, but the Sa_{O_2} often is not adversely affected.

Fiberoptic Bronchoscopy and Tracheobronchial Anatomy

- Trachea and main carina (Figure 3-2)
  - ▲ The main carina normally has a sharp bifurcation.
  - ▲ The membranous trachea is posterior and has a flat appearance.
  - ▲ The anterior trachea is arc-shaped and has visible rings.
- Right mainstem bronchus and secondary carina (Figure 3-3)
  - ▲ On the right is the orifice of the RUL.
  - ▲ On the left is the origin of the right bronchus intermedius.
- RUL bronchus and segmental bronchi (Figure 3-4)
  - ▲ Unique trifurcation includes apical, anterior, and posterior segments.

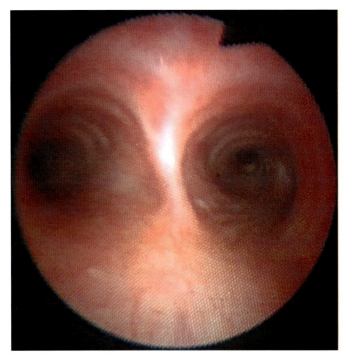

Figure 3-2. View of the main carina shows the arc-shaped rings of the anterior trachea above and the posterior membranous trachea below.

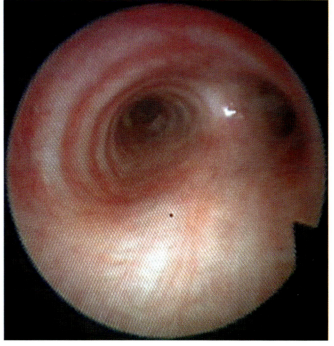

Figure 3-3. The right mainstem bronchus has the orifice of the right upper lobe to the right and the origin of the bronchus intermedius to the left.

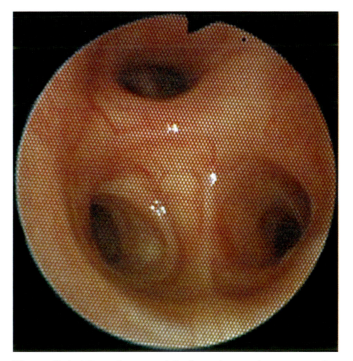

Figure 3-4. The right upper lobe bronchus is characteristically trifurcated into three segments.

- Right bronchus intermedius and bifurcation into the right middle lobe (RML) and right lower lobe (RLL) (Figure 3-5)
  - ▲ RML has a slightly smaller lumen and two bronchial segments.
  - ▲ RLL has a larger lumen with one superior and four basal segments.
- Left mainstem bronchus, carina, and bifurcation into the left upper lobe (LUL) and left lower lobe (LLL) (Figure 3-6)
  - ▲ The LUL and LLL are approximately equal in size.
- Left lower lobe (Figure 3-7)
  - ▲ One superior segment and three (usually) or four basal segments
- Left upper lobe (Figure 3-8)
  - ▲ Upper division has three segments.
  - ▲ Lingula has two segments, usually immediately visible.

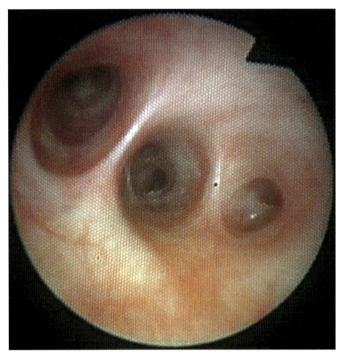

Figure 3-5. In the right bronchus intermedius, the right middle lobe orifice is smaller, and the right lower lobe orifice typically has a flat septum separating the superior segment from the basal segments.

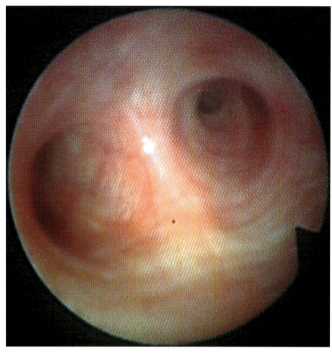

Figure 3-6. In the left mainstem bronchus, the left upper lobe and left lower lobe bronchi are approximately equal in size.

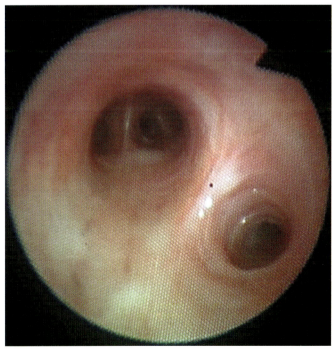

Figure 3-7. The left lower lobe bronchus has one superior segment and three (sometimes four) basal segments.

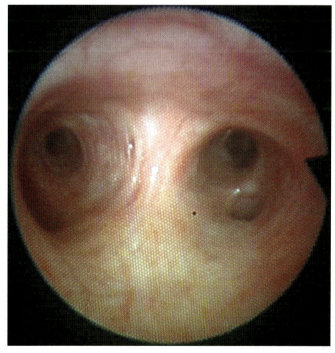

Figure 3-8. In the left upper lobe bronchus, the upper division has three segments, and the lingula has two segments.

- ◆ Optimally placed right DLT
  - ▲ View through bronchial lumen: RUL takeoff is visible through the aperture in the DLT at the end of the white line (Figure 3-9).
  - ▲ View through tracheal lumen: blue rim of the distal cuff is visible at right of carina (Figure 3-10).

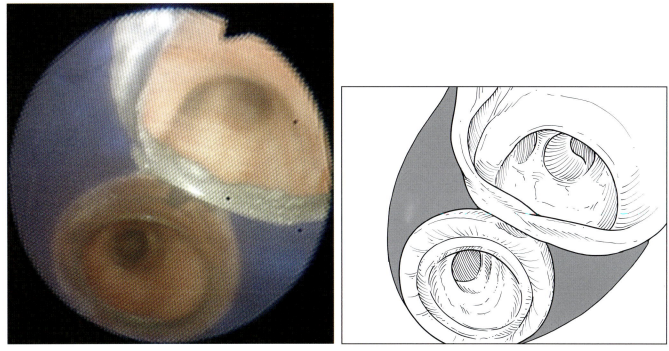

Figure 3-9. View through the bronchial lumen of an optimally placed right double-lumen endotracheal tube shows the takeoff of the right upper lobe orifice through the aperture at the end of the white line.

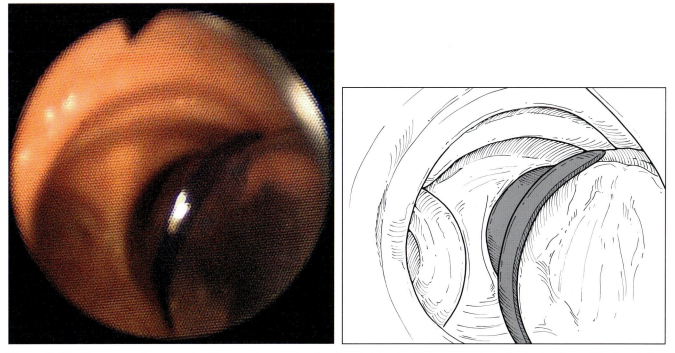

Figure 3-10. View through the tracheal lumen of an optimally placed right double-lumen endotracheal tube shows the rim of the distal cuff to the right of the carina.

- Optimally placed left DLT
  - ▲ View through bronchial lumen: left mainstem carina and the LUL and LLL bronchi are visible (Figure 3-11).
  - ▲ View through tracheal lumen: blue rim of the distal cuff is visible at left of carina (Figure 3-12).

Induction, Maintenance, and Emergence from Anesthesia

- All medication choices are geared toward prompt emergence from anesthesia and extubation in the operating room whenever possible.
- Reduce FIO_2 in any patient who has received neoadjuvant chemotherapy or radiation therapy to reduce the risk of hyperoxic lung injury; oxygen saturation of 86% to 90% is acceptable during one-lung ventilation.
- Minimize intravenous fluid administration to reduce the risk of postexpansion pulmonary edema.

Induction

- Avoid benzodiazepines in geriatric patients or any patient with borderline respiratory function.
- Propofol is well tolerated by most patients, although we often use reduced doses; etomidate is appropriate for patients with compromised cardiac function or hypovolemia.
- Keep narcotic doses low to avoid postoperative respiratory depression; 100 to 150 mcg of fentanyl is sufficient for many cases.
- Intubation is usually accomplished with nondepolarizing muscle relaxants; rocuronium has the advantages of rapid onset and minimal histamine release.

Maintenance

- Clamp the tracheal lumen of the DLT well before surgical entry to the thorax to allow the lung time to deflate; confirm tube placement with FOB after lateral positioning, and suction the operated lung as necessary.
- Dexamethasone (8 to 10 mg IV) helps to reduce vocal cord edema, diminish airway reactivity, and prevent postoperative nausea.
- Desflurane is a useful inhaled agent because it can be rapidly titrated on and off, and it acts as an effective bronchodilator. Desflurane reduces hypoxic pulmonary vasoconstriction but not to a clinically significant degree.
- Propofol infusion may be helpful, especially for rigid bronchoscopy in which an air leak may limit the use of inhaled agents.
- Maintain normothermia with fluid warming (especially if transfusion is necessary) and use of a forced-air warming blanket for the lower body.

Intraoperative Issues and Caveats

- Short-lived fluctuations in blood pressure are common because of variations in the level of surgical stimulus, mechanical pressure on the heart or great vessels, and relatively dry fluid status.
- Pharmacologic support of low blood pressure is better than giving large quantities of crystalloid. Hypertension can be managed acutely with small doses of propofol or esmolol; use longer-acting antihypertensive agents only with caution until surgery ends.
- Intraoperative arrhythmias are often secondary to instrumentation and resolve when manipulation is stopped.
- Diltiazem (20 mg IV) may be given slowly to reduce the incidence of postoperative atrial fibrillation in patients undergoing lobectomy or pneumonectomy, particularly if the pericardium is entered.

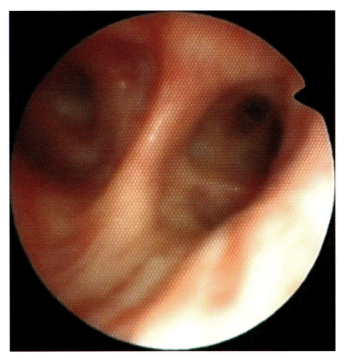

Figure 3-11. View through the bronchial lumen of an optimally placed left double-lumen endotracheal tube shows the left upper lobe and left lower lobe bronchi.

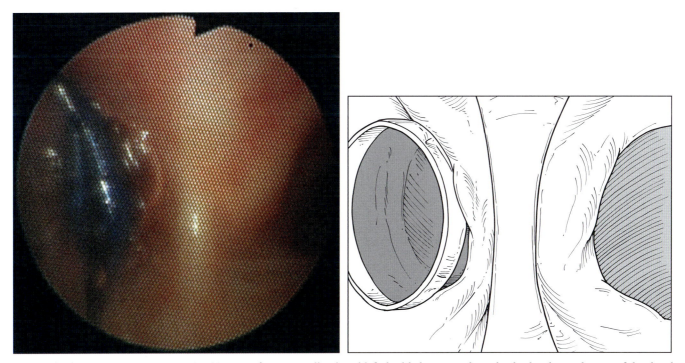

Figure 3-12. View through the tracheal lumen of an optimally placed left double-lumen endotracheal tube shows the rim of the distal cuff to the left of the carina.

- Avoid overdosing with muscle relaxants; thoracic patients may be at risk for prolonged muscle relaxant effects due to Eaton-Lambert syndrome, myasthenia gravis, steroid-induced myopathy, or chronic debilitation.

Ventilation Parameters

- During one-lung ventilation, reduce the tidal volume (V_T) to 5–6 mL/kg.
- Monitor to ensure a peak airway pressure (PAP) of less than 35 cm H_2O and a plateau pressure of less than 25 cm H_2O.
- Apply PEEP up to 5 cm H_2O except for patients with chronic obstructive pulmonary disease (COPD).
- Adjust the respiratory rate to maintain a normal Pa_{CO_2}.
- Use pressure-controlled ventilation for patients with reduced lung compliance or other risk factors for acute lung injury:
  - ▲ Idiopathic pulmonary fibrosis
  - ▲ Restrictive or obstructive lung disease with reduced D_{LCO} or FEV_1
  - ▲ Prior chemotherapy or radiation therapy
  - ▲ Alcohol abuse
  - ▲ Blood transfusion (transfusion-related acute lung injury [TRALI])
  - ▲ Exposure to drugs associated with pulmonary toxicity, such as amiodarone, bleomycin, cyclophosphamide, tocainide, crack cocaine, and heroin
  - ▲ Underlying connective tissue disorder, such as rheumatoid arthritis, scleroderma, lupus, Wegener's disease, and Goodpasture's syndrome
  - ▲ Hyperoxia: consider reducing F_{IO_2} whenever feasible after initial denitrogenation.

Emergence

- Reinflate the operative lung gradually; manual ventilation is the best means of controlling airway pressure.
- Consider allowing the patient to resume spontaneous ventilation during closure of the subcutaneous tissue and skin.
- The use of pressure support with or without synchronized intermittent mandatory ventilation (SIMV) facilitates spontaneous ventilation and lung reinflation.
- Ensure that muscle relaxation is completely reversed!
- Extubate patients awake in the semi-sitting position if they are obese or were difficult to intubate.
- Consider deep extubation in the lateral position for selected patients (e.g., normal weight, easy airway); this has the advantage of reducing cough, bronchospasm, hypertension, and tachycardia.
- Add ketorolac (30 mg IV) near the end of the case for patients with normal renal function and coagulation parameters.
- Lidocaine (50 to 100 mg IV) may help the patient tolerate the endotracheal tube until extubation.
- Many patients benefit from bronchodilator therapy immediately on arrival to the postanesthesia care unit (PACU).

Procedure-Specific Pearls and Pitfalls

Mediastinoscopy

- Significant blood loss rarely occurs but can be massive and can require median sternotomy for control.
- Place the pulse oximeter sensor and arterial catheter (if used) on the patient's right. If the mediastinoscope occludes the brachiocephalic artery, diminished blood flow to the right arm can be recognized promptly and the surgeon alerted so that the duration of reduced flow to the right carotid artery can be minimized.

Thymectomy for Myasthenia Gravis
- Avoid muscle relaxants if possible.
- Adequate intubating conditions may be achieved with a combination of propofol and deep anesthesia with inhaled agents (i.e., desflurane or sevoflurane).

Bilateral Thoracic Sympathectomy
- Bilateral thoracic sympathectomy is frequently performed on healthy patients for hyperhidrosis.
- A single-lumen tube suffices, and respiration is suspended during the key portions of surgical exposure while CO_2 is insufflated to decompress the lung.
- Monitor bilateral upper extremity temperatures for confirmation of sympathectomy.

Esophagectomy
- Depending on the site of the lesion, the patient may require right video-assisted thoracic surgery (VATS) or right thoracotomy in addition to laparotomy.
- The left side of the neck must be left free if a cervical anastomosis is planned.
- Hypotension is common during mediastinal dissection of the esophagus and may require pharmacologic support; some surgeons request dopamine infusion routinely.
- Maintain normal temperature and acid-base status; these patients require generous hydration.
- Prolonged hypotension or hypovolemia may contribute to ischemia of the esophageal anastomosis.

Pleurodesis and Decortication
- Pleurodesis and decortication are often undertaken in very ill patients with metastatic cancer, chronic pleural effusion, empyema, or hemothorax.
- Anticipate substantial intraoperative blood loss during decortication, especially if the pleural peel is old.
- These patients are at high risk for postoperative mechanical ventilation due to their underlying disease processes.

Bilateral Lung Volume Reduction Surgery
- Lung volume reduction surgery is recommended only for patients with severe, refractory COPD.
- Bronchodilator and steroid therapy should be optimized preoperatively.
- Instruct the patient in the use of pursed-lip breathing after surgery to augment pulmonary function by supplying auto-PEEP.
- A thoracic epidural catheter should be placed before surgery unless there is a contraindication (see "Postoperative Analgesia").
- Gentle induction works best, with reduced propofol dosing, a nondepolarizing muscle relaxant, and an inhaled agent for bronchodilation.
- Highly compliant lungs with bleb formation reach excessive tidal volumes easily; avoid aggressive mask ventilation during induction.
- Maintain pressure-controlled ventilation with initial peak inspiratory pressure (PIP) settings of 12 to 14 cm H_2O (preferred). PIP greater than 20 cm is rarely necessary.
- Allow higher than normal Pco_2 (i.e., permissive hypercapnia) with slower inspiratory and expiratory cycling of the ventilator to reduce the risk of barotrauma and air trapping. Oxygenation is seldom a problem.
- Lung deflation often requires FOB-directed suctioning.
- Reinflation of the first lung should be accomplished by manual ventilation with pressures of less than 20 cm, gradually increasing each breath until the lung is expanded. Although the surgeon may request higher pressure to test the suture line, it is important to avoid causing another bleb to rupture.

- Assess suture line leaks by using a volume meter attached to the anesthesia circuit. At a reasonable PIP, measure the difference between inspiratory and expiratory volumes. Too great a difference implies that the suture line must be inspected for a leak. Some air leak is to be expected; the amount varies according to the patient's lung volumes.
- As operation begins on the second side, the ventilated lung is the previously reduced lung. Compliance is often decreased, and a lower tidal volume must be tolerated to avoid excessive PIP.
- Check for excessive air leak on the second side as described previously.
- Extubate the patient in a semi-sitting position when awake and following commands; encourage the use of pursed-lip breathing.
- Order bronchodilator treatment to be started immediately on arrival to the PACU.

Postoperative Analgesia

Analgesia for Routine Thoracoscopic Cases

- In our institution, less than 5% of thoracoscopic cases convert to open thoracotomy, and we do not place epidural catheters for routine single-lung VATS procedures.
- The surgeons infiltrate the skin with local anesthesia before incision and often perform thoracic intercostal nerve blocks from T2 to T11 before wound closure.
- Ketorolac is a useful adjunct.
- The PACU nursing staff plays a vital role in titrating narcotic analgesia. Too little can cause the patient to splint and refuse to cough due to pain; too much can easily result in carbon dioxide retention. Small incremental doses work best, such as hydromorphone (0.2 to 0.5 mg IV) or fentanyl (25 to 50 mcg IV).

Thoracic Epidural Analgesia

- We place epidural catheters preoperatively in patients undergoing open thoracotomy, pneumonectomy, lung volume reduction surgery, bilateral VATS, and rib or chest wall resection.
- About 5% of video-assisted lobectomies are scheduled as possible open thoracotomies due to previous neoadjuvant radiation therapy or chemotherapy, Pancoast tumor, chest wall involvement, or the need for sleeve resection; these patients receive epidural catheters.
- Epidural placement before induction of general anesthesia produces improved analgesia because the epidural can be activated before the conclusion of surgery.
- The epidural catheter is usually inserted at the mid-thoracic level. Placement at a more cephalad level does not block pain from the chest tube insertion sites.
- In the event of unanticipated conversion of VATS to open thoracotomy, some anesthesiologists place an epidural catheter before emergence from anesthesia, with minimal or reversed neuromuscular blockade. Others prefer to awaken the patient and insert the epidural in the PACU.
- Anesthesiologists disagree about whether it is ever justifiable to insert a thoracic epidural catheter in an unconscious adult patient who cannot report pain or paresthesia.
- We make limited use of the epidural catheter during surgery except to give a test dose of local anesthetic and a loading dose of 2.5 to 4 mg of preservative-free morphine. A fully activated epidural increases the risk of intraoperative hypotension.
- Because fluid administration is kept to a minimum for most thoracic patients, especially those undergoing pneumonectomy, blood pressure may need support with a low-dose infusion of phenylephrine for the first 24 hours.

- Near the conclusion of surgery, we administer epidural fentanyl (50 to 100 mcg) with 0.25% bupivacaine or 1% lidocaine with 1:200,000 epinephrine (4 to 6 mL). A continuous infusion is started after the patient arrives in the PACU, usually consisting of fentanyl (5 to 10 mcg/mL) and bupivacaine (0.05% to 0.0625%) at 3 to 6 mL/hr.
- Communication with PACU staff and the pain management service is essential for continuity of care during the postoperative period.

CHAPTER 4

APPLIED ANATOMY

Cynthia S. Chin and Scott J. Swanson

Introduction

Anatomy of the thoracic cavity is constant regardless of the surgical approach, but the vantage point is different with the use of open surgery or minimally invasive surgery. When performing video-assisted thoracoscopic surgery (VATS), the surgeon must understand the anatomy as viewed from the videoscope and as seen through a thoracotomy. This chapter describes the techniques of exposure for the major anatomic structures in the thorax.

Right Upper Lobectomy

Anterior Hilum

- **Exposure:** Retract the lung posteriorly.
- Aim the thoracoscope anteriorly and medially.
- The phrenic pedicle travels in a superoinferior direction on the superior vena cava and heart (Figure 4-1). Identify this structure so that it is not inadvertently injured in dissection of the superior pulmonary vein (SPV) (Figure 4-2). Using blunt dissection, the phrenic nerve and its vessels can be swept anteriorly away from the pulmonary vein (Figure 4-3).
- The important structures are the SPV, which is most anterior; the right pulmonary artery, which is posterior and often superior to the SPV; and the right upper lobe bronchus, which is the most posterior structure and often can be identified after the SPV and the truncus anterior branch of the pulmonary artery are divided (Figure 4-4).

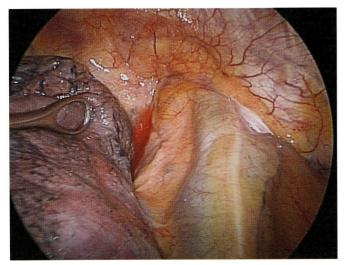

Figure 4-1. The right phrenic nerve crosses the first part of the subclavian artery as it enters the thoracic cavity. It travels along the superior vena cava as it goes inferiorly toward the diaphragm.

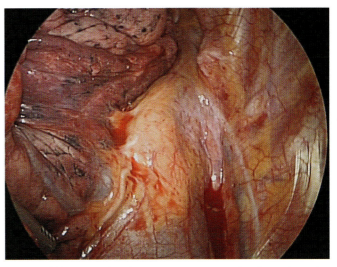

Figure 4-2. The right phrenic nerve courses closely to the right hilum. The right upper lobe is retracted posteriorly, and the phrenic nerve can be seen traveling across the superior pulmonary vein.

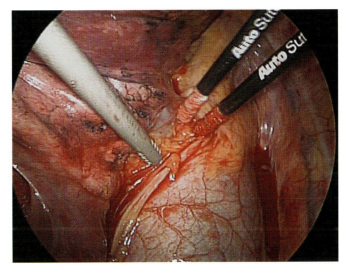

Figure 4-3. The right phrenic nerve is bluntly dissected from the superior pulmonary vein. Using two endokittners, the phrenic nerve can be swept away from the superior pulmonary vein to avoid inadvertent injury during ligation of the vein for a right upper lobectomy.

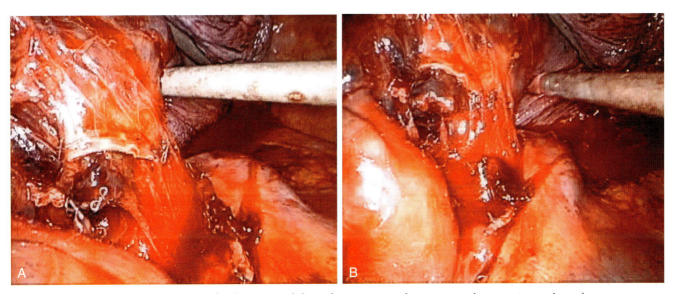

Figure 4-4. A, In the superior aspect of right anterior hilum, the superior pulmonary vein lies anterior to the pulmonary artery, which lies anterior to the bronchus of the right upper lobe. **B,** The anterior aspect of the right upper lobe bronchus can be visualized after the superior pulmonary vein and the truncus anterior branch of the pulmonary artery are ligated.

• With retraction of the lung inferiorly from the posterior incision, the azygous vein can be identified passing to the superior vena cava from a posterior direction (Figure 4-5). It is positioned just superior to the truncus anterior branch of the pulmonary artery and the right mainstem bronchus. It should be dissected bluntly away from these structures. Mobilizing the azygous vein allows complete node dissection (Figure 4-6). If there are any problems with visualization of the nodes, the vein can be readily divided with the endovascular stapler.

Posterior Hilum

• **Exposure:** Retract the lung anteriorly.
• Aim the thoracoscope posteriorly.
• After opening the posterior mediastinal pleura with the harmonic scalpel or cautery device, you can see the subcarinal space with the right mainstem bronchus and bronchus intermedius traveling in an oblique direction toward the lung (Figure 4-7).
• The azygous vein travels up the posterior chest wall before turning anterior at the level of the carina (Figure 4-8). With gentle blunt dissection, free the vein from the right mainstem bronchus.

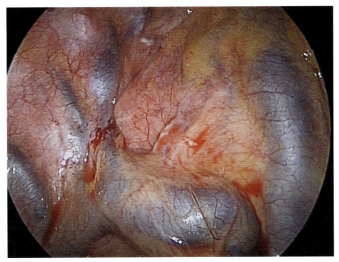

Figure 4-5. The azygous vein travels anteriorly at the level of the carina over the superior portion of the right hilum to join the superior vena cava. It is close to the right upper lobe bronchus and the truncus anterior branch of the pulmonary artery at this location.

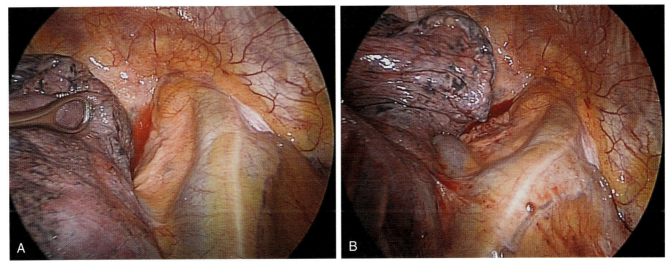

Figure 4-6. Level 4R paratracheal nodes lay posterior to the confluence of the azygous vein and superior vena cava. Diseased lymph nodes may adhere to one or both structures, and care must be taken to avoid injury to these vessels. **A,** shows a lymph node anterior to vagus nerve. **B,** shows scar at junction of azygous vein and SVC.

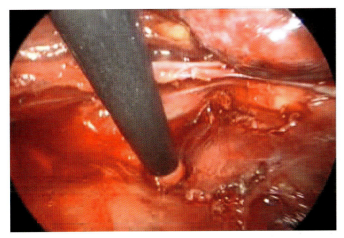

Figure 4-7. In the right subcarinal space, the right mainstem bronchus emerges from under the azygous vein just before the takeoff of the right upper lobe bronchus.

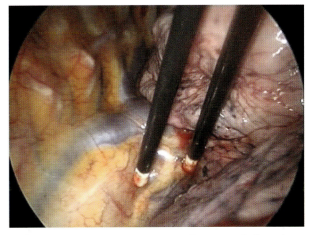

Figure 4-8. The azygous vein travels superiorly lateral to the right border of the thoracic vertebral bodies.

- During the subcarinal node dissection, the entire subcarinal space is well visualized. The esophagus lies anterior to the left mainstem bronchus (Figure 4-9). After the nodes are completely resected, hemostasis is straightforward and can be accomplished with surgical cellulose and pressure. Use thermal energy discretely to avoid injury to the membranous right mainstem bronchus or the esophagus.
- Sweeping mediastinal pleura up toward the lung permits visualization of the right upper lobe bronchus taking off at a 90-degree angle from the right mainstem bronchus (Figure 4-10).
- The thoracic duct lies posterior to the esophagus and is rarely an issue, although with extensive node dissection in the subcarinal space, significant thoracic duct radicals can be disrupted. Use clips on any lymphatic vessels of significant size (>2 mm).
- Extensive paratracheal node dissection extends to the apex of the right chest. Identify the right subclavian artery and vein (Figure 4-11). Avoid extensive thermal dissection in this region to avoid injury to the right recurrent nerve. Medially and anteriorly, the left innominate vein joins the right innominate vein to form the superior vena cava (Figure 4-12). It should be identified during the high paratracheal node dissection. The pericardium can be seen at the base of the paratracheal node dissection after the nodes are removed.

Right Middle Lobectomy

- **Exposure:** Retract the lung posteriorly.
- Aim the thoracoscope anteromedially.
- The phrenic nerve courses in an inferior direction over the base of the middle lobe pulmonary vein (Figure 4-13). Similar to the dissection for the upper lobectomy, bluntly sweep away the nerve to avoid injury to it. The middle lobe pulmonary vein usually drains into the left atrium with the superior pulmonary vein but can drain separately or, rarely, with the inferior pulmonary vein. The middle lobe vein is composed of two segmental veins, with one anterior to the other or, less commonly, with one superior to the other.

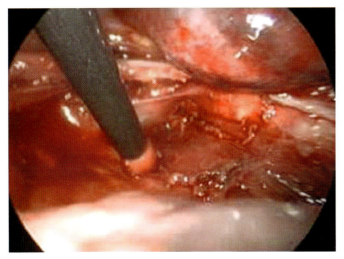

Figure 4-9. The left mainstem bronchus is visualized from the right hemithorax during dissection of the subcarinal space.

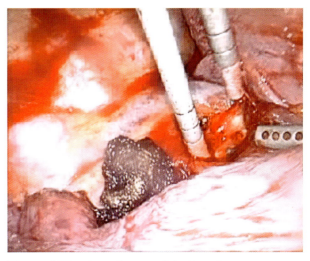

Figure 4-10. The right upper lobe bronchus (posterior aspect) is best visualized after the mediastinal pleura is swept toward the lung.

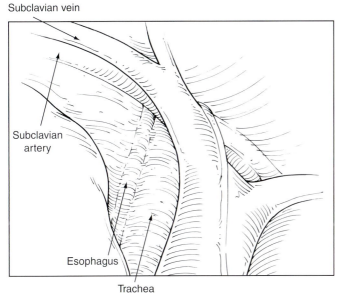

Figure 4-11. The right subclavian artery and vein can be seen in the apex of the right hemithorax.

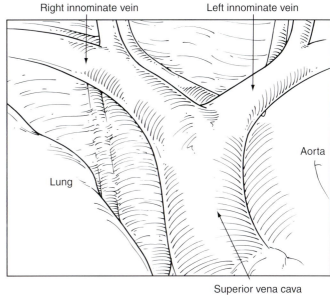

Figure 4-12. The left innominate vein crosses the mediastinum to join the right innominate vein to form the superior vena cava.

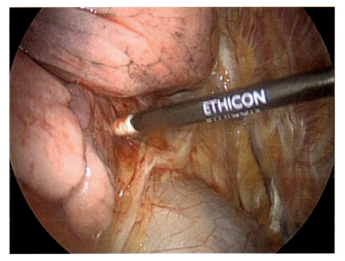

Figure 4-13. The middle lobe vein usually drains into the superior pulmonary vein.

- Unlike with the upper lobe, the bronchus sits posterior to the vein with the middle lobe pulmonary arteries posterior to the bronchus or slightly superior to the bronchus (Figure 4-14). This relationship is important because after dividing the middle lobe vein, the next step is to divide the middle lobe bronchus. In passing the right-angle clamp around the bronchus, be aware of the artery's location to avoid injuring it with the clamp. The artery may be swept away from the bronchus bluntly before passing the clamp.
- Because the middle lobe is an anterior structure, the entire dissection is focused on the anterior aspect of the chest, and this is the easiest lobe to resect.

Right Lower Lobectomy

- **Exposure:** Retract the lung anteriorly.
- Aim the thoracoscope posteriorly.
- The initial view for the lower lobectomy involves the posterior hilum (Figure 4-15). You should understand the relationships among the inferior pulmonary vein, the ongoing pulmonary artery, and lower and middle bronchi. Dissection on the superior and inferior border of the inferior pulmonary vein from the posterior hilum defines this vein and identifies the lower lobe bronchus and ongoing pulmonary artery, which lie immediately superior to the superior border of the inferior vein. The diaphragm may impede the view and may be retracted with an endokittner through the camera port or with an EndoStitch device.
- Identify the superior segmental pulmonary artery, which is the most posterior branch of the right pulmonary artery (Figure 4-16). After dividing this branch, you can divide the basilar trunk without concern.
- Consider the relationship between the lower lobe bronchus and middle lobe bronchus (Figure 4-17), and identify the takeoff of the middle lobe bronchus to avoid kinking the middle lobe bronchus in dividing the lower lobe bronchus. The anesthesiologist can perform bronchoscopy before the division of the lower lobe bronchus to ensure there is no distortion of the middle lobe bronchus.
- Avoid injury to the phrenic nerve in the region of the inferior pulmonary vein because it can sometimes pass very close to the inferior border of the vein before arborizing on the central tendon of the diaphragm (Figure 4-18). Exuberant use of the cautery can cause an injury in this location.

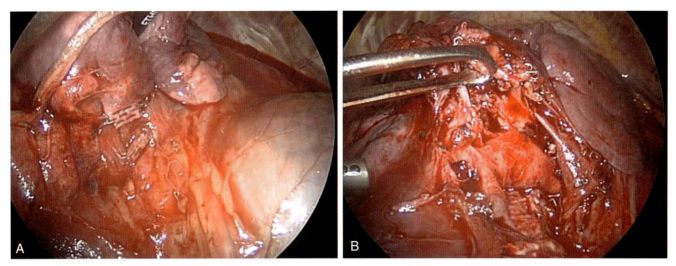

Figure 4-14. A, The middle lobe bronchus lies just deep to the divided middle lobe vein seen in the picture. **B**, The allis clamp is holding the divided middle lobe bronchus. Behind is the ongoing pulmonary artery.

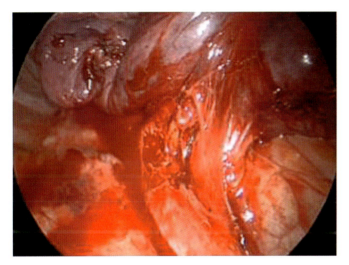

Figure 4-15. Posterior view of the lower lobe.

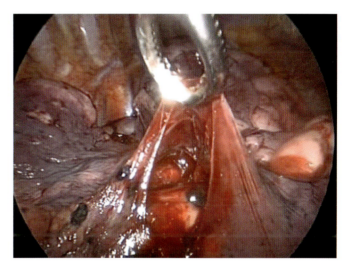

Figure 4-16. The pulmonary artery enters the fissure at the confluence of the minor and major fissures. The superior segmental artery is posterior to the basilar artery.

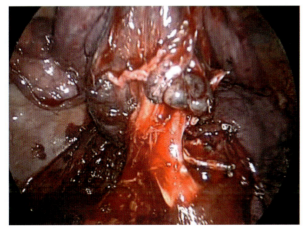

Figure 4-17. The middle lobe bronchus travels from the bronchus intermedius to the middle lobe through the anterior portion of the major fissure.

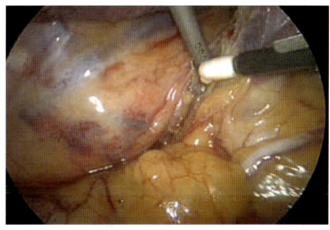

Figure 4-18. The phrenic nerve can lie very close to the inferior border of the inferior pulmonary vein. As the inferior pulmonary ligament is divided, pay careful attention to this relationship.

Left Upper Lobectomy

- **Exposure:** Retract the lung posteriorly and inferiorly.
- Aim the thoracoscope anteriorly and medially.
- Notice several anatomic structures: the aortic arch, the subclavian artery (Figure 4-19), the aortic pulmonary window (Figure 4-20), the aortic phrenic nerve (Figure 4-21), the left vagus nerve with its accompanying recurrent laryngeal nerve (Figure 4-22), and the esophagus.

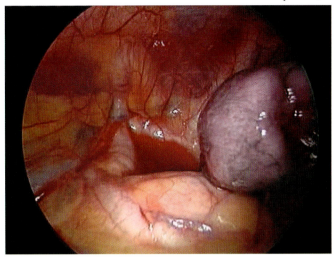

Figure 4-19. Aortic arch. The left subclavian artery travels from the aortic arch to a position under the clavicle in the left hemithorax.

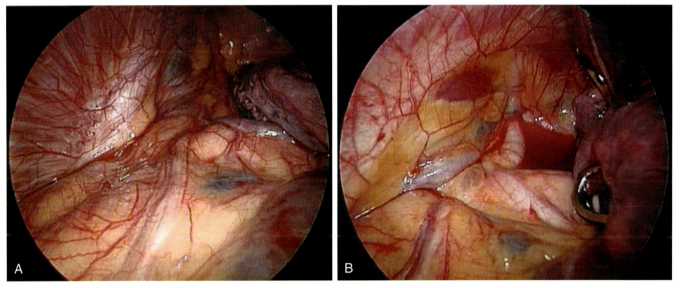

Figure 4-20. The aortic pulmonary window can be visualized only from the left chest. A level 5 lymph node can be sampled by careful dissecting in this area. **A** and **B** are two different views of the lymph nodes in the aortic pulmonary window.

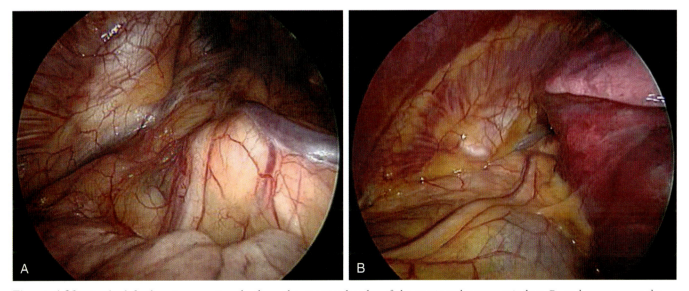

Figure 4-21. A, The left phrenic nerve travels along the anterior border of the aortic pulmonary window. **B,** and passes onto the pericardium

(Continued)

- The best way to assess level 5 (see Figure 4-20) and level 6 lymph nodes (Figure 4-23) is from a left thoracoscopic approach at the outset of a lobectomy. Bluntly sweep these nodes away from the recurrent laryngeal nerve at its takeoff from the vagus nerve at the level of the aortic arch. During proximal node dissection superior to the arch, be aware of the vagus nerve (Figure 4-24) because any injury at this level affects the recurrent laryngeal nerve, which takes off distal to this level. Medially at this level, the left innominate vein passes obliquely toward the midline to form the superior vena cava.
- Similar to the right side, the phrenic nerve courses from superior to inferior along the anterior hilum of the lung and should be swept away bluntly at the time of the dissection of the upper pulmonary vein and branches of the pulmonary artery to the upper lobe (see Figure 4-21).
- For left-sided pulmonary surgery, the surgeon must have a good understanding of the left pulmonary artery. It is short, and if there are any issues with dissection of the branches of the pulmonary artery, the surgeon should obtain proximal control before any bleeding occurs. Tamponade bleeding with a sponge stick through the anterior incision, although this makes it difficult to gain proximal control because of the short vessel length. If using an intrapericardial approach to the left main pulmonary artery, be careful not to compress or impede the outflow track of the right ventricle.

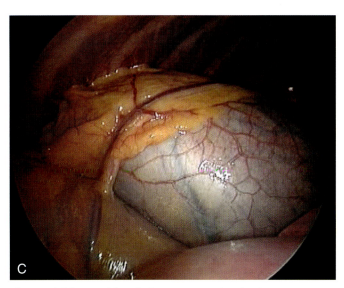

Figure 4-21. cont'd C, before entering the diaphragm. Pay careful attention when lysing adhesions between the left lung and the pericardium.

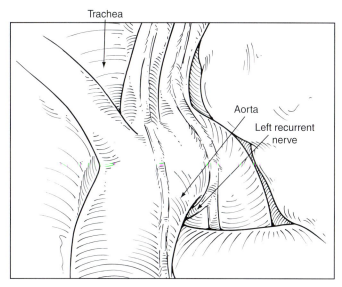

Figure 4-22. The left vagus nerve travels anterior to posterior, crossing over the aortic arch, and it travels along the posterior hilum before entering the abdomen with the esophagus. The left recurrent nerve is given off by the vagus at the level of the aortic arch.

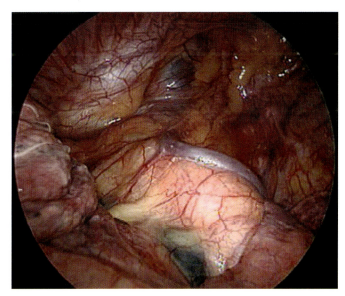

Figure 4-23. Level 6 lymph nodes can be visualized by retracting the left upper lobe anteriorly and slightly inferiorly.

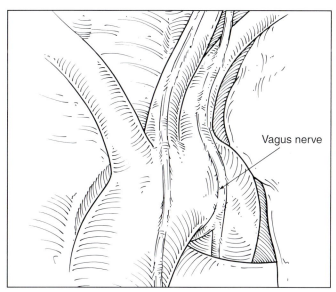

Figure 4-24. Injury to the superior portion of the vagus nerve proximal to the aortic arch affects the function of the left recurrent laryngeal nerve.

- In posterior hilar dissection, identify the posterior pulmonary arterial branches, and dissect out the level 10, 7, 8, and 9 lymph nodes. The esophagus is deep to the aorta at this level (Figure 4-25). The longitudinal muscle fibers are easy to identify. In dissecting the level 7 lymph nodes from the left side, gently retract the aorta and esophagus posteriorly to open up the subcarinal space (Figure 4-26). If there is bleeding in this region during dissection, the best initial approach is to pack the area with surgical cellulose to permit a better visualization of the source, which usually is a nodal artery that can be clipped or cauterized. Spare the vagus nerve, which passes from a superior to inferior direction in the posterior direction just medial to the aorta and along the esophagus, by sweeping it posteriorly along the surface of the aorta. Some of the branches to pulmonary hilum may be divided sharply to facilitate this.

Left Lower Lobectomy

- **Exposure:** Retract the lung anteriorly.
- Aim the thoracoscope posteriorly.
- The diaphragm obscures the view of the inferoposterior hilum. Retract it with an Endokittner or EndoStitch device in the posterior aspect of the central tendon (Figure 4-27).
- After the inferior pulmonary ligament is released, the inferior vein is exposed. It is identified by the almost constant appearance of a level 9 lymph node at its inferior border (Figure 4-28). When this is observed, the vein is immediately superior to it. Because the esophagus can be adherent inferior and posterior to the vein, keep the dissection just inferior to the lower edge of the lung when releasing the ligament.

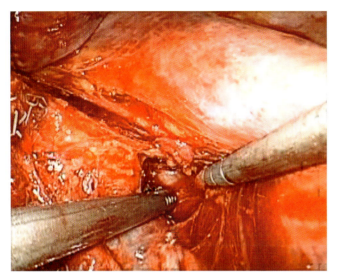

Figure 4-25. For most of its thoracic course, the esophagus lies just to the right of the aorta. At the level of the diaphragm, it takes a more anterior position in relation to the aorta.

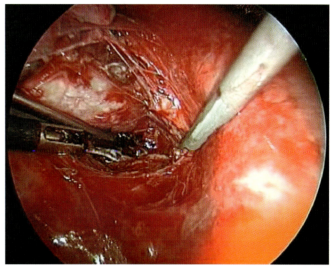

Figure 4-26. The aorta and underlying esophagus must be gently retracted posteriorly to access the subcarinal space posteriorly. The vagus nerve can be retracted posteriorly to avoid injury. Some vagal branches to the lung may require ligation. Irritation or injury of the vagus nerve during surgery can cause bradycardia intraoperatively and constipation postoperatively.

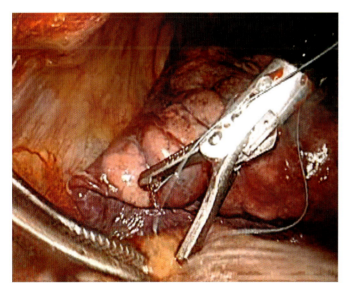

Figure 4-27. The endostitch is used to place a 2-0 tevdek suture into the central tendon of the diaphragm to be used for inferior retraction and optimal visualization of the inferior pulmonary hilum.

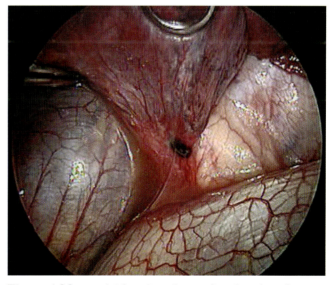

Figure 4-28. Level 9 lymph nodes are found in the inferior pulmonary ligament at the inferior border of the inferior pulmonary vein.

- Similar to the procedure for the right side, you should understand the relationships among the inferior pulmonary vein, the bronchus, and the pulmonary artery where it passes from its posterior location into the fissure. It is easier to identify the left pulmonary artery entering the fissure than the right, because its course is more direct into the fissure (Figure 4-29) and the middle lobe does not obscure its path. The takeoff of the superior segmental pulmonary artery is easy to identify (Figure 4-30). Often, the vagus nerve courses very close to the posterior aspect of the left lower lobe bronchus and vein. You can sweep it posteriorly to preserve it.
- The anatomy of the left lower lobe is consistent, and there is no middle lobe on the left, making this perhaps the easiest of the major lobes to resect using a VATS.

Esophageal Resection

- **Exposure:** Retract the lung anteriorly.
- Aim the thoracoscope posteriorly.
- The esophagus runs from the thoracic inlet to the esophageal hiatus in a direct superoinferior direction (Figure 4-31).

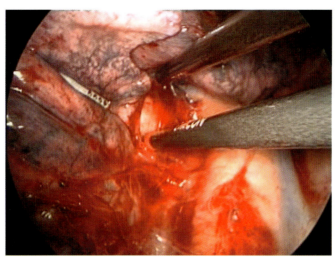

Figure 4-29. The left pulmonary artery passes posteriorly to the left upper lobe bronchus. The left pulmonary artery is the most posterior structure in the left hilum.

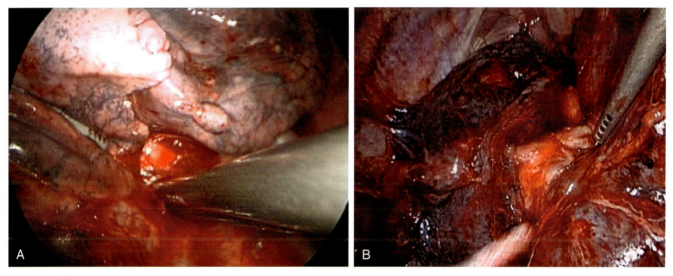

Figure 4-30. Arterial branches to the left upper lobe are the most variable. Including the first branch of the left pulmonary artery, there can be two to eight arteries supplying the left upper lobe. The left lower lobe is similar to the right lower lobe, with a superior segmental and basilar arterial supply. **A,** The proximal left pulmonary artery is seen during the initial dissection of the anterior hilum. **B,** The distal left pulmonary artery, in the fissure, is seen with tip of the suction irrigator at the level of the proximal superior segmental artery.

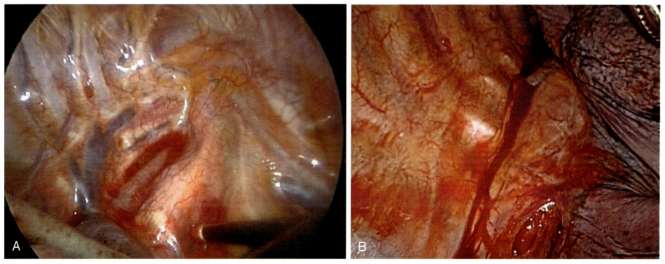

Figure 4-31. A right hemithorax view of the thoracic esophagus shows the superior portion **A,** traveling under the azygous

(Continued)

- It usually is best to approach the esophagus from the right side when resecting it above its midportion because of the aortic arch on the left side (Figure 4-32).
- The airway lies anterior to the esophagus, and the aorta is located posteriorly. The thoracic duct runs posterior to the esophagus beginning at the esophageal hiatus, and it crosses to the left side at the level of the carina (T4). The vagal nerves run on the left and right sides of the esophagus.
- You can dissect the esophagus circumferentially using blunt dissection and electrocautery or harmonic energy.
- Because of the proximity of the esophagus to the right and left mainstem bronchi, the surgeon should avoid injury to the membranous airways by staying in an appropriate plane and not straying with the dissection when using electrocautery.
- When dissecting the esophagus from the aorta, use clips or the harmonic scalpel to secure the aortoesophageal branches. The more inferior branches usually are larger and require more attention. In this location, there may be large thoracic duct branches that should be similarly clipped. If there is any question about this approach, prophylactic use of an EndoStitch device is reasonable and can be accomplished by suturing all tissue between the aorta and azygous vein at the most inferior aspect of the chest.

Thymectomy

- **Exposure:** not applicable.
- Aim the thoracoscope medially from the right side.
- The thymus gland is a midline structure located in the anterior mediastinum. It extends into the neck and can be accessed from the right side of the chest.
- The phrenic nerve outlines the lateral extent of the dissection (Figure 4-33). The left phrenic nerve can be identified from the right side in most cases. All tissue medial to this, including that in the anteroposterior window, must be removed. If visualization is difficult, a left-sided camera port may be placed.
- The right internal mammary vein drains into the right innominate vein and can be divided just before its entrance into the innominate vein to open up the space between the anterior and superior mediastinum.
- Two to three draining thymic veins drain from the body of the thymus into the left innominate vein, running in an inferosuperior direction (Figure 4-34). They should be divided between clips or with the harmonic scalpel.
- The pericardium outlines the posterior extent of the dissection.
- The diaphragm outlines the inferior extent of the dissection, and all associated fat should be removed with the thymus to remove any ectopic thymic tissue. The cervical poles of the thymus can be seen extending into the neck and can be teased out from the right VATS approach. Draining vessels can be clipped or cauterized.

Sympathetic Chain

- **Exposure:** Retract the lung anteriorly.
- Direct the thoracoscope posteriorly.
- The sympathetic chain runs from the thoracic inlet to the posterior diaphragmatic hiatus in a relatively straight superoinferior direction.
- For sympathectomy, identify the chain at the head of the second rib (Figure 4-35), and divide it.
- The first rib is usually difficult to visualize, but it is delineated by its short and characteristic C shape.

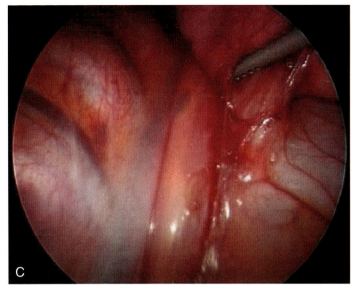

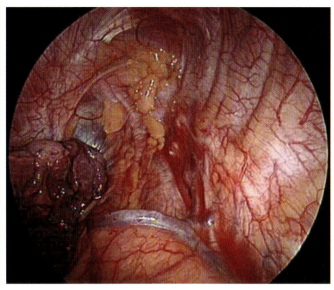

Figure 4-31. cont'd B, and passing through the diaphragm **C,** on its way to the abdomen.

Figure 4-32. The thoracic esophagus can be visualized in the left hemithorax above the aortic arch. However, at the level of the arch, the esophagus is obscured. Distal to this point, the esophagus lies to the right of the aorta until just before it enters the diaphragm, where it lies anterior to the aorta.

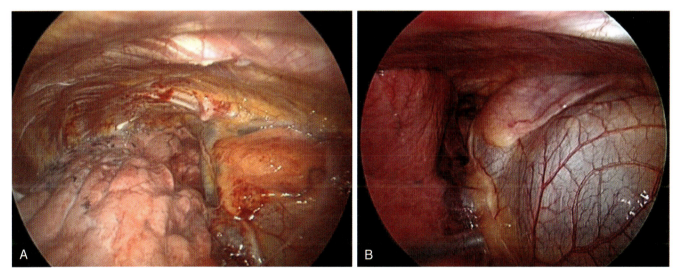

Figure 4-33. In the anterior mediastinum, the phrenic nerves mark the lateral extent of dissection during a thymectomy.

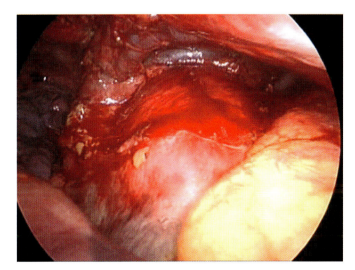

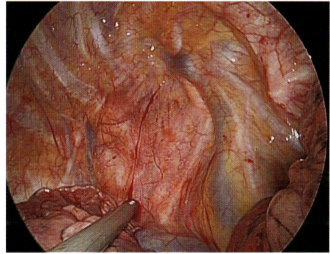

Figure 4-34. The thymus has two or three veins that drain into the left innominate vein.

Figure 4-35. The right sympathetic chain travels along the posterior chest wall. The sympathetic ganglia run just below the corresponding rib heads. For example, the T2 ganglion runs between the second and third rib heads.

CHAPTER 5

WEDGE RESECTION AND BRACHYTHERAPY FOR LUNG CANCER—VIDEO 5

Robert J. McKenna, Jr. and Robert J. McKenna, III

Introduction

Compared with a lobectomy, wedge resection carries a three to five times greater risk of local recurrence and has a lower survival rate.[1] The standard of practice for the surgical treatment of lung cancer is a lobectomy, but because some patients cannot physiologically tolerate a lobectomy, an alternative is needed. Traditional external beam radiation can have the same negative impact on pulmonary function as a lobectomy. Wedge resection with localized radiation (i.e., brachytherapy) has been developed as better alternatives. Because preliminary series have shown very good results, an intergroup, randomized trial (ACOSOG Z4032) has been undertaken to evaluate the long-term benefits of brachytherapy for reducing the risk of local recurrence.

Santos and colleagues described one approach to brachytherapy. They embedded iodine 125 sutures in a Vicryl mesh that was subsequently secured to the surface of the lung at the margin of the resection.[2] This provided a radiation dose of 100 Gy to a depth of 5 mm. The brachytherapy group had a lower local recurrence rate (19% versus 2%, $P =$ .0001).[2] There were no adverse effects related to the placement of the brachytherapy mesh, including no radiation pneumonitis, no implant migration or implant-related morbidity, and no compromise of pulmonary function when comparing preoperative and postoperative values. A concern regarding that approach is the radiation exposure for intraoperative personnel and for the patient's visitors. An alternative approach with afterload catheters appears to have similar results.[3] Both approaches are described in this chapter.

Key Points

- Perform wedge resection with the goal of a 2-cm margin around the tumor.
- Place mesh embedded with radiation seeds or afterload catheters on the surgical margin.

Criteria

Indications
- Non–small cell lung cancer or pulmonary metastasis
- Small (<3 cm), peripheral masses
- Zubrod performance status score of 0, 1, or 2
- Forced expiratory volume in 1 second (FEV$_1$) <50% predicted
- Diffusing capacity of the lung for carbon monoxide (D$_{LCO}$) <50% predicted
- Partial pressure of carbon dioxide (Paco$_2$) >45 mm Hg
- Patients not candidates for lobectomy (e.g., pulmonary hypertension, severe medical illnesses)

Contraindications
- Prior ipsilateral thoracic surgery
- Prior ipsilateral thoracic radiation
- Pregnancy

Approach to Wedge Resection and Brachytherapy

Step 1. Incisions
- Make the standard incisions (see Figure 1-2 in Chapter 1).
- The utility incision (incision 3) should be only 2 cm long, and incision 4 is not needed.

Step 2. Wedge Resection
- **Exposure:** Retract the lung posteriorly and slightly inferiorly.
- Aim the thoracoscope anteriorly with the 30-degree lens pointed toward the apex of the chest.
- The goal of resection is a 2-cm gross margin around the tumor.
- Ring forceps hold the lung 1 to 2 cm inferior to the tumor and in a line between the mass and the thoracoscope. Hold the parenchyma so that the stapler easily slides across the lung tissue. You can compress the lung parenchyma below the tumor, in the anticipated path of the stapler, to facilitate passage of the stapler across the lung.
- Introduce the stapler through incision 1 for the wedge resection (Figure 5-1).
- After firing the stapler enough times to transect lung tissue beyond the tumor, perform a final firing of the stapler through incision 3 to perpendicularly transect and separate the specimen from the remainder of the lung (Figure 5-2).

Step 3. Afterload Catheters
- **Exposure:** Retract the lung posteriorly and slightly inferiorly.
- Aim the thoracoscope anteriorly with the 30-degree lens pointed posteriorly.
- Place three 3-0 polydioxanone sutures (PDS) on the staple line (Figure 5-3).
- Pass the afterload catheter through the sutures.
- Tie the sutures in place. This usually can be accomplished with extracorporeal knot tying. A finger through incision 3 secures the knots (Figure 5-4).
- A large clip is placed on the staple line closest to where the tumor was resected. This helps with the subsequent planning by the radiation therapist.

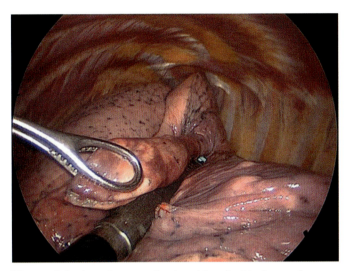

Figure 5-1. A wedge resection is achieved with the stapler through incision 1.

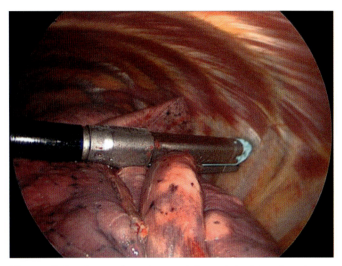

Figure 5-2. The stapler is inserted through incision 3 and crosses the lung to be resected.

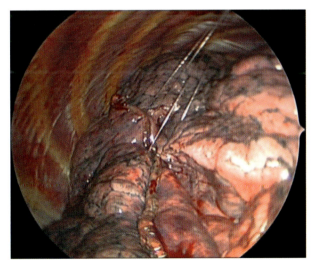

Figure 5-3. Sutures are placed to hold the brachytherapy afterload catheters.

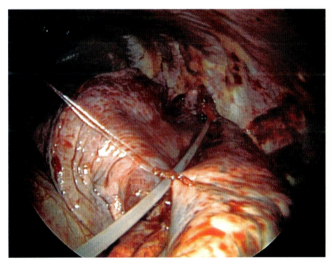

Figure 5-4. The first brachytherapy catheter is sewn in place with the 3-0 PDS suture.

Step 4. Additional Afterload Catheters
- **Exposure:** Retract the lung posteriorly and slightly inferiorly.
- Aim the thoracoscope anteriorly with the 30-degree lens pointed posteriorly.
- Secure additional catheters parallel to and 1 cm away from the staple line (Figure 5-5).

Step 5. Catheters through the Chest Wall
- **Exposure:** Retract the lung posteriorly and slightly inferiorly.
- Aim the thoracoscope anteriorly with the 30-degree lens pointed posteriorly.
- Bring the catheters through the anteroinferior chest wall.
- Pass the catheters through a metallic button that is secured to the skin. Crimp the metal with a clamp to prevent the afterload catheters from falling out. If the metal is crimped too tightly, the radioactive seeds cannot readily be passed through the catheters.

Step 6. Postoperative Care
- Brachytherapy is high-dose radiation (HDR); a robot passes the seeds into the afterload catheters to avoid radiation exposure by health care personnel.
- Treatment schedule
  - ▲ Monday: operation
  - ▲ Tuesday: computed tomography (CT) scan for planning
  - ▲ Tuesday through Friday: twice-daily radiation treatments
  - ▲ Friday: brachytherapy catheters and chest tube removed in anticipation of patient discharge

Alternative Approach to Wedge Resection and Brachytherapy

Step 1. Wedge Resection
- The wedge resection or segmentectomy is performed in the same manner through the same incisions.

Step 2. Mesh with Iodine 125
- Brachytherapy mesh with the 125I seeds is commercially available (Johnson & Johnson, Somerville, NJ).
- Each seed has an activity of 0.4 to 0.6 mCi.

Step 3.
- **Exposure:** Retract the lung posteriorly and slightly inferiorly.
- Aim the thoracoscope anteriorly with the 30-degree lens pointed posteriorly.
- Pass the mesh through incision 1.
- Place it on the surface of the lung, centered on the staple line closest to where the tumor had been, and suture it to the lung.

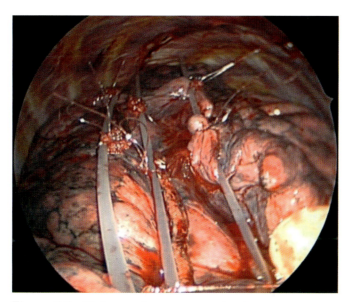

Figure 5-5. All three catheters are sewn in place.

Radiation Safety After Iodine 125 Seed Implantation

Intraoperative Considerations (Not Afterload Catheter Method)
- There is minimal radiation risk for operating room personnel and family members due to the 1-cm range of the radiation.
- The radiation therapist handles the 125I seeds with long instruments (>15 cm) to minimize contact.
- Dose rate at 1 mis recorded, and the operating room is surveyed to ensure that there are no loose or lost sources.

Postoperative Considerations
- Postoperatively, the patient is in an isolation room throughout the hospitalization.
- No pregnant women are allowed in the area of the patients during or after seed placement.

Discharge Instructions per ACOSOG Z4032 Protocol
- Children should not sit on the patient's lap for more than 5 minutes per day for 6 months after 125I seed implantation.
- Patients should be at least 3 feet away from any pregnant woman for 3 months after seed implantation.
- There are no restrictions regarding tableware, dishes, linen, clothing, and toilet facilities.
- Touching, shaking hands, or kissing does not make others radioactive.

References
1. Ginsberg RJ, Rubinstein LV: Randomized trial of lobectomy versus limited resection for T1N0 lung cancer, *Ann Thorac Surg* 60:615–621, 1995.
2. Santos R, Colonias A, Parda D, et al: Comparison between sublobar resection and 125 I brachytherapy following sublobar resection in high risk patients with stage 1 non-small cell lung cancer, *Surgery* 134:691–697, 2003.
3. McKenna RJ Jr, Mahtabifard A, Yap J, et al: Wedge resection and brachytherapy for lung cancer in patients with poor pulmonary function, *Ann Thorac Surg* 85:S733–S736, 2008.

Lobectomies and Pneumonectomies

CHAPTER 6

VIDEO–ASSISTED LOBECTOMY: GENERAL CONSIDERATIONS

Robert J. McKenna, Jr.

Introduction

A lobectomy performed as video-assisted thoracic surgery (VATS) should be a standard, anatomic resection, just as a lobectomy performed through a thoracotomy.

Criteria

Indications and contraindications for a VATS-type lobectomy are given in Table 6-1. Most lobectomies can be performed by VATS. We perform more than 90% of our lobectomies by VATS. The ribs are not spread. Larger tumors (5 to 8 cm) can be resected through a 5- to 6-cm incision if the rib is shingled posteriorly. Because tumors larger than 8 cm in diameter take up so much space in the chest, it is difficult to manipulate the lobe to perform the dissection, and these large tumors require a thoracotomy.

Relative contraindications are factors that may make the procedure difficult or unsafe. Dissection of abnormal nodes adherent to the vessels, preoperative chemotherapy, and preoperative radiation therapy may mandate a thoracotomy. However, we have performed 18 bronchial sleeve resections, and we usually can perform lobectomies[1] and full node dissections after neoadjuvant chemotherapy for stage III lung cancers.[2,3]

Absolute contraindications are factors that make a VATS-type resection almost impossible. If the tumor is too large, it cannot fit through the small incision used in VATS. Tumors attached to the chest wall, including Pancoast tumors, require a thoracotomy and rib resection. Combined chemotherapy and radiation therapy usually make enough scar tissue around the vessels that a thoracotomy is needed to complete the nodes dissection and to safely dissect around vessels.

Video-Assisted Lobectomy

- Usually work from anterior to posterior.
- To ensure safety, identify the vessels. Expose the vessels to ensure they are not accidentally transected or injured and to position the stapler for safe and anatomic resections.
- It is safest to dissect on named structures. Paradoxically, staying closer to the pulmonary vessels and bronchi greatly reduces the chances of inadvertent injury.
- The fissures are completed with staples to reduce air leaks. Dissection is not performed in the fissure to expose the vessels.

TABLE 6-1.   Indications and Contraindications for Video-Assisted Lobectomy

INDICATIONS	RELATIVE CONTRAINDICATIONS	CONTRAINDICATIONS
Stage 1 lung cancer	Tumor 5-8 cm in diameter	Tumors >8 cm in diameter
Tumor <6 cm	Preoperative irradiation	Mediastinal invasion
Benign disease (e.g., bronchiectasis)	Preoperative chemotherapy	Surgeon discomfort
	Sleeve resections	
	Chest wall invasion	

Postoperative Care After Video-Assisted Thoracic surgery

- Postoperative care is streamlined after VATS.[4] No routine laboratory tests or radiographs are used. Laboratory tests are performed if there are arrhythmias, fevers, or other specific indications.
- The chest drainage system is attached to an intravenous line pole so that the patients can more easily ambulate and get to the bathroom and to prevent the drainage system from falling over. The drainage system is not placed on suction because randomized studies have shown prolonged air leaks when suction is applied.[5] Suction is applied to the drainage system for patients with increased postoperative drainage, such as extensive adhesions that were lysed or significant subcutaneous emphysema.
- Chest radiographs are needed for patients with dyspnea, hypoxia, or significant subcutaneous emphysema and for fever workup. Chest radiographs are not performed after removal of chest tubes, unless the patients develop significant dyspnea, hypoxia, or subcutaneous emphysema.

Advantages of Video-Assisted Lobectomy

- Although there are no large multi-institutional, randomized trials comparing VATS and thoracotomy for lobectomy, the mounting data show many advantages for the VATS approach.
- After VATS, patients have a shorter hospital stay,[2,3] possibly less morbidity and mortality,[2,3,6] less pain,[6] better pulmonary function,[7,8] and less cost. Frail patients tolerate it better,[9] and patients recover faster.[10]
- Because patients recover faster after VATS than after a thoracotomy, they have a better chance of receiving full doses of their adjuvant chemotherapy.[11,12]

Learning About Video-Assisted Lobectomy

◆ Attend a VATS-type lobectomy course, usually more than once. The initial course can help you understand the basic approach. During additional courses, more subtle details of the procedure that were missed during an introductory course may become clear.
◆ Read book chapters and atlases.
◆ Study videos.
◆ Consult with a new associate who has experience with the procedure.
◆ Transition gradually from a posterolateral incision to a muscle-sparing incision to VATS. With the muscle-sparing incision, you move to the front of the patient. The incision is in the location of the utility incision (incision 3) for a video-assisted lobectomy. It starts at the edge of the latissimus muscle and extends anteriorly. The latissimus is not mobilized or cut. A few fibers of the serratus are separated. The intercostal muscles are cut from the internal mammary vessels to the spine. Dissect the hilum of the lung anteriorly to posteriorly, as for a VATS-type lobectomy. Do some of the dissection while looking at a monitor. As you make the transition from open surgery to VATS, make the incision smaller, and do not spread the ribs.

References

1. Mahtabifard A, Fuller CB, McKenna RJ Jr: VATS sleeve lobectomy, *Ann Thorac Surg* (in press).
2. McKenna RJ Jr, Houck W, Fuller CB: Video-assisted thoracic surgery lobectomy: experience with 1100 cases, *Ann Thorac Surg* 81:421–426, 2006.
3. Onaitis MW, Petersen RP, Balderson SS, et al: Thoracoscopic lobectomy is a safe and versatile procedure: experience with 500 consecutive patients, *Ann Surg* 244:420–425, 2006.
4. McKenna RJ Jr, Mahtabifard A, Fuller CB: Fast tracking after VATS pulmonary resection, *Ann Thorac Surg* (in press).
5. Cerfolio RJ, Bass C, Katholi C: Prospective randomized trial compares suction versus water seal for air leaks, *Ann Thorac Surg* 71:1613–1617, 2001.
6. Whitson BA, Groth SS, Duval SJ, et al: Surgery for early-stage non-small cell lung cancer: A systemic Review of the video-assisted thoracoscopic surgery versus thoracotomy approaches to lobectomy, *Ann Thorac Surg* 86:2008–2018, 2008.
7. Nomori H, Ohtsuka T, Horio H, et al: Difference in the impairment of vital capacity and 6-minute walking after a lobectomy performed by thoracoscopic surgery, an anterior limited thoracotomy, an antero-axillary thoracotomy, and a posterolateral thoracotomy, *Surg Today* 33:7–12, 2003.
8. Nakata M, Saeki H, Yokoyama N, et al: Pulmonary function after lobectomy: video-assisted thoracic surgery versus thoracotomy, *Ann Thorac Surg* 70:938–941, 2000.
9. Demmy TL, Curtis JJ: Minimally invasive lobectomy directed toward frail and high-risk patients: a case-control study, *Ann Thorac Surg* 68:194–200, 1999.
10. Demmy TL, Plante AJ, Nwogu CE, et al: Discharge independence with minimally invasive lobectomy, *Am J Surg* 188:698–702, 2004.
11. Nakajima J, Takamoto S, Kohno T, Ohtsuka T: Costs of videothoracoscopic surgery versus open resection for patients with lung carcinoma, *Cancer* 89(Suppl):2497–2501, 2000.
12. Petersen RP, Pham D, Burfeind WR, et al: Thoracoscopic lobectomy facilitates the delivery of chemotherapy after resection for lung cancer, *Ann Thorac Surg* 83:1245–1249, discussion 1250, 2007.

CHAPTER 7

PNEUMONECTOMY—VIDEO 7

Robert J. McKenna, Jr.

Introduction

A pneumonectomy can be performed with video-assisted thoracic surgery (VATS), and the specimen usually fits through the same size of incision as is used for a VATS-type lobectomy, depending on the size and location of the lesion. Usually, a large central tumor is not appropriate for VATS because of its involvement of the mediastinal structures. The surgeon must ensure that the tumor is not amenable to a sleeve resection, which sometimes is difficult to ascertain by a VATS approach. Therefore, it is the rare pneumonectomy that is best handled by VATS.

Approach to Video-Assisted Pneumonectomy

Order of Operative Steps

The order of the steps for a pneumonectomy is as follows: removal of level 10 nodes on the right or level 6 and 5 nodes on the left, superior pulmonary vein (SPV), inferior pulmonary vein (IPV), pulmonary artery, subcarinal nodes, and mainstem bronchus.

Key Points

- Remove the lymph nodes early to define the anatomy and make the procedure safer.
- Remove the level 5 nodes to expose SPV and the pulmonary artery.
- Use a noncutting stapler on the pulmonary artery in case the device misfires.
- A good subcarinal node dissection ensures the mainstem bronchus is stapled very close to the carina.
- Use an open stapler, such as the TA 30 (Covidien Inc., Mansfield, MA) or TX 30 (Ethicon Endosurgery, Cincinnati, OH) for the bronchus. Put the pin down, and pull the lung through the stapler to get the stapler as close as possible to the carina.

 ## Left Pneumonectomy (Video 7-1)

Step 1. Level 5 and 6 Node Dissection on the Left

- **Exposure:** Retract the lung posteriorly and slightly inferiorly.
- Aim the thoracoscope anteriorly with the 30-degree lens pointed posteriorly.
- Dissect at the inferior aspect of the SPV. Lift the inferior aspect of the fat with a ring forceps. Use Metzenbaum scissors at the junction of the fat and the pericardium.

- Pull the fat inferiorly and posteriorly to expose the phrenic nerve. Metzenbaum scissors incise the pleura, just posteriorly to the phrenic nerve. Rotate the Metzenbaum scissors clockwise to see the nerve well and avoid cutting it.
- Incise the pleura along the superior aspect of the SPV and the vein from the apex of the lung. Continue over the superior aspect of the hilum, because this mobilizes the anterior trunk of the artery (Figure 7-1).
- Dissect on named structures (usually blunt dissection) along SPV, pulmonary artery, pericardium, and aorta. Lift the adipose and lymphatic tissue with a ring forceps through incision 3. Dissect with the Metzenbaum scissors or the Yankauer suction catheter through incision 1.
- Carefully identify the phrenic, vagus, and recurrent laryngeal nerves.

Step 2. Left Superior Pulmonary Vein

- **Exposure:** Retract the lung posteriorly and slightly inferiorly.
- Aim the thoracoscope anteriorly with the 30-degree lens pointed posteriorly.
- With the Metzenbaum scissors, dissect the superior aspect of the SPV (Figure 7-2).
- Lift the SPV with a ring forceps (Figure 7-3), and with the Metzenbaum scissors or the Yankauer suction catheter through incision 1, dissect under the SPV. The bronchus is directly behind the vein.
- With DeBakey forceps through incision 3, lift the soft tissue between the SPV and the pulmonary artery.
- Using Metzenbaum scissors through incision 1, dissect on the superior aspect of the SPV.
- A right-angle clamp through incision 1 moves inferiorly to superiorly around the SPV (Figure 7-4). Blunt dissection with the right-angle instrument can be performed several times to mobilize the SPV. Progress of the dissection can be seen better if the 30-degree lens is rotated to look from posterior to anterior and if the SPV is lifted with a ring forceps or a pickup.
- Be careful when lifting pulmonary vessels. The vein should be held with a good purchase to minimize the chances of injury. A small purchase on a pulmonary vessel may tear the surface of the vessel.
- When the right-angle clamp has nearly passed around the SPV, look for the tip of the right-angle instrument on the superior aspect of the SPV. This can be seen better if the 30-degree lens is rotated to look from anterior to posterior.
- Spread widely with the right-angle clamp to create a large tunnel that easily allows passage of the stapler from incision 4.
- Staple the vein (Figure 7-5). Have a ring forceps in the chest through incision 3 as the stapler fires. The staple line may leak, and a ring forceps in the chest can control the bleeding.

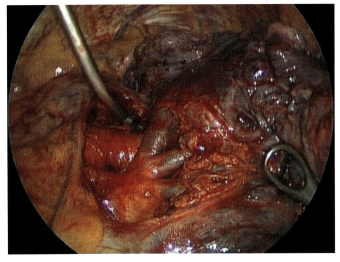

Figure 7-1. Dissection along the pulmonary vein over the superior aspect of the hilum.

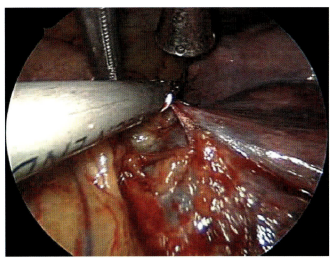

Figure 7-2. Dissection along the superior aspect of the left superior pulmonary vein.

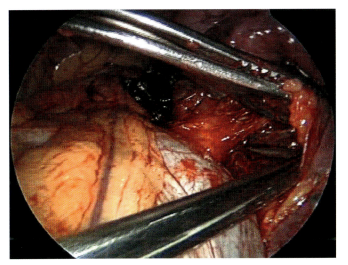

Figure 7-3. Dissection of the inferior aspect of the left superior pulmonary vein.

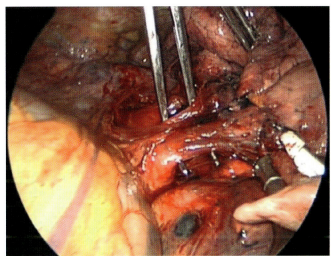

Figure 7-4. Right-angle clamp around the left superior pulmonary vein.

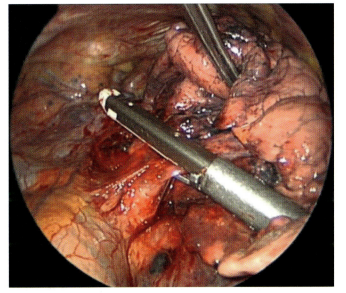

Figure 7-5. Stapling the left superior pulmonary vein.

Step 3. Left Inferior Pulmonary Vein

* **Exposure:** Retract the lung directly toward the apex of the chest.
* Aim the thoracoscope anteriorly with the 30-degree lens pointed posteriorly.
* The diaphragm can be retracted with the curve of the Yankauer suction and the tip of the suction pointed toward the inferior pulmonary ligament.
* A ring forceps through incision 3 retracts the lung directly toward the apex of the chest.
* Extension of the electrocautery through incision 1 takes down the inferior pulmonary ligament.
* Remove level 9 and 8 nodes with electrocautery.
* Retract the lung slightly posteriorly to dissect bluntly between the IPV and the SPV. This can be accomplished quickly with the Yankauer suction. The vein from the superior segment can be seen.
* Retract the lung anteriorly. Metzenbaum scissors through incision 1 incise the pleura posterior to the IPV. Dissection continues along the pericardium. A lymph node located posterior and superior to the IPV can be held with a ring forceps from incision 4. Removal of that node greatly facilitates IPV mobilization (Figure 7-6).
* Metzenbaum scissors, the Yankauer suction, or a right-angle clamp through incision 1 or 3 passes around the IPV (Figure 7-7).
* A stapler through incision 1 or 3 transects the IPV (Figure 7-8).

Step 4. Left Subcarinal Node Dissection

* **Exposure:** Retract the lung directly anteriorly.
* Aim the thoracoscope anteriorly with the 30-degree lens pointed posteriorly.
* Retract the lung directly anteriorly with ring forceps.
* Use Metzenbaum scissors through incision 1 to cut the pleura along the bronchus and just anterior to the vagus nerve.
* Blunt dissection with the Yankauer suction or the Metzenbaum scissors through incision 1 begins on the surface of the pericardium. A ring forceps from incision 4 holds the soft tissue in the subcarinal space. The esophagus and the vagus nerve constitute the posterior border for the dissection. There is a tendency to dissect toward the esophagus, but the dissection should be away from the esophagus and toward the bronchus.
* A ring forceps from incision 4 can retract the esophagus posteriorly. This exposes the subcarinal nodes. When they are completely removed, the right and the left mainstem bronchi are seen clearly (Figure 7-9).

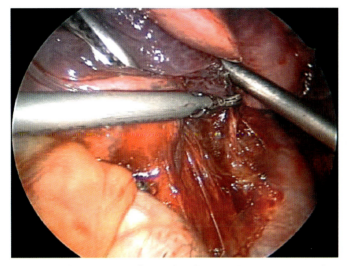

Figure 7-6. Exposure of the left inferior pulmonary vein and removal of the posterior node.

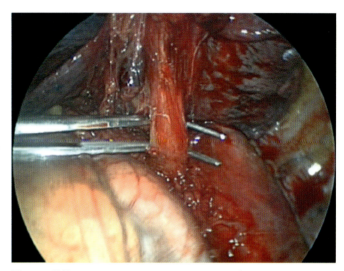

Figure 7-7. Right-angle clamp around the left inferior pulmonary vein.

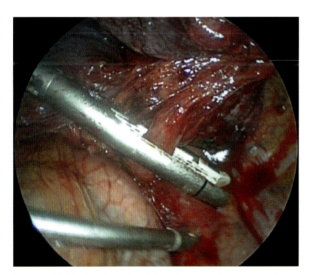

Figure 7-8. Stapling the left inferior pulmonary vein.

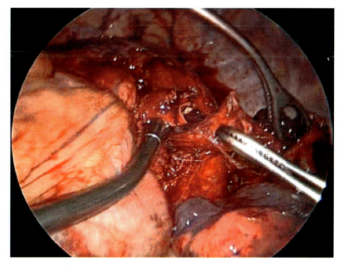

Figure 7-9. Empty subcarinal space.

Step 5. Left Pulmonary Artery

- **Exposure:** Retract the lung posteriorly and slightly inferiorly.
- Aim the thoracoscope anteriorly with the 30-degree lens pointed posteriorly.
- The inferior aspect of the pulmonary artery is well exposed after the SPV and IPV have been transected. Perform blunt dissection with a Yankauer suction or Metzenbaum scissors through incision 3 between the pulmonary artery and the bronchus (Figure 7-10).
- The superior aspect of the pulmonary artery is well exposed after the nodes have been dissected. Perform blunt dissection with a Yankauer suction or Metzenbaum scissors through incision 3 into the aortopulmonary window.
- Through incision 3, a right-angle clamp passes around the pulmonary artery after the blunt dissection has nearly completely mobilized the artery.
- Use an open stapler, such as the Covidien TA 30 or Ethicon TX 30 for the artery. Put the pin down, and pull the lung through the stapler to position the stapler (Figure 7-11).
- Placement of an additional stapler more distally on the artery can prevent back bleeding when the artery is transected with scissors or a scalpel through incision 3.

Step 6. Left Mainstem Bronchus

- **Exposure:** Retract the lung posteriorly and slightly inferiorly.
- Aim the thoracoscope anteriorly with the 30-degree lens pointed posteriorly.
- Subcarinal node dissection has already mobilized the posterior aspect of the mainstem bronchus.
- Anteriorly, the bronchus needs to be mobilized from the pericardium. Accomplish this with blunt or sharp dissection through incision 3.
- Aortopulmonary node dissection mobilizes the superior aspect of the mainstem bronchus.
- Use an open stapler, such as the TA 30 (US Surgical, Norwalk, Conn) or Ethicon TX 30 for the bronchus. Put the pin down, and pull the lung through the stapler to position the stapler as close as possible to the carina.
- Cut the bronchus with Metzenbaum scissors or a scalpel through incision 3.

Step 7. Lung Removal

- **Exposure:** Retract the lung posteriorly and slightly inferiorly.
- Aim the thoracoscope anteriorly with the 30-degree lens pointed posteriorly.
- Pull the lung with a ring forceps to the bottom of the chest to create a space for the removal bag. A ring forceps through incision 3 places the base of the Lapsac bag (Cook, Bloomington, Indiana) at the apex of the chest.
- Two ring forceps through incision 3 hold the bag open.
- A ring forceps from incision 4 or 1 pushes the lung into the bag. This usually takes several steps. When the lung is partially placed in the bag, the ring forceps pinches the lung, and the ring forceps that was holding the lung grabs a lower purchase on the lung and again pushes it into the bag.

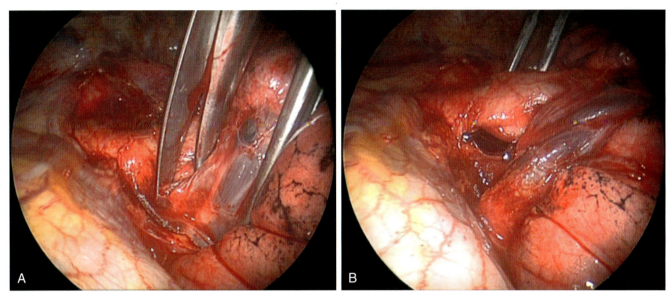

Figure 7-10. Dissection between the left main pulmonary artery and the bronchus. **A,** Scissors dissect the main pulmonary artery. **B,** Right angle passes around the main pulmonary artery.

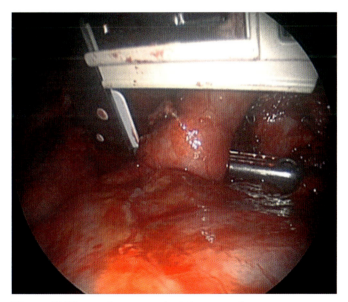

Figure 7-11. Stapler across the left main pulmonary artery.

Right Pneumonectomy (Video 7-2)

Step 1. Level 10 Node Dissection
- **Exposure:** Retract the lung posteriorly and slightly inferiorly.
- Aim the thoracoscope anteriorly with the 30-degree lens pointed posteriorly.
- The Metzenbaum scissors and the DeBakey pickups incise the pleura just posterior to the phrenic nerve and from the SPV to the azygous vein.
- Incise the pleura along the inferior aspect of the azygous vein. To see this area well, retract the lung slightly more inferiorly. The 30-degree lens and the thoracoscope are rotated slightly clockwise (Figure 7-12).
- Incise the pleura on the superior aspect of the IPV and the vein from the apex of the right upper lobe.
- Lift the fat and level 10 nodes to dissect along the pericardium, vessels, and the right mainstem bronchus.
- When the nodes have been removed, through incision 3, apply a Yankauer suction tip or the Metzenbaum scissors bluntly along the superior aspect of the right main pulmonary artery.
- Transection of the azygous vein by an endoscopic stapler through incision 1 or 4 opens the space for subsequent mobilization of the main pulmonary artery and for level 2 and 4 node dissection.

Step 2. Right Superior Pulmonary Vein
- **Exposure:** Retract the lung posteriorly and slightly inferiorly.
- Aim the thoracoscope anteriorly with the 30-degree lens pointed posteriorly.
- With the Metzenbaum scissors or the Yankauer suction catheter through incision 1, bluntly dissect between the SPV and the IPV (Figure 7-13).
- Lift the SPV with a ring forceps or DeBakey pickups. With the Metzenbaum scissors or the Yankauer suction catheter through incision 1, dissect under the SPV. The artery is directly behind the vein.
- With DeBakey forceps through incision 3, lift the soft tissue between the SPV and the pulmonary artery.
- With Metzenbaum scissors through incision 1, dissect on the superior aspect of the SPV.
- A right-angle clamp through incision 1 runs inferiorly to superiorly around the SPV (Figure 7-14). Blunt dissection with the right-angle clamp can be performed several times to mobilize the SPV. Progress of the dissection can be seen better if the 30-degree lens is rotated to look from posterior to anterior and the SPV is lifted with a ring forceps or a pickup.
- Be careful when lifting pulmonary vessels. The vein should be held with a good purchase to minimize the chances of injury. Inadequate purchase on a pulmonary vessel may tear the surface of the vessel.
- When the right-angle clamp has nearly passed around the SPV, look for the tip of the right-angle instrument on the superior aspect of the SPV. This can be seen better if the 30-degree lens is rotated to look from anterior to posterior.
- Spread widely with the right-angle clamp to create a large tunnel that easily allows passage of the stapler from incision 4.
- Staple the vein (Figure 7-15). Have a ring forceps in the chest through incision 3 as the stapler fires. If the staple line leaks, use a ring forceps to apply pressure and control the bleeding.

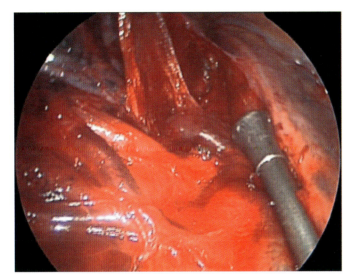

Figure 7-12. Dissection for the level 10 nodes.

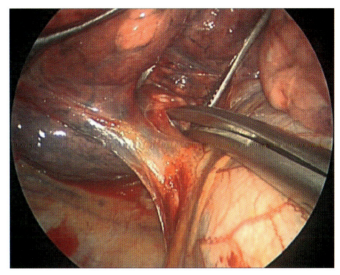

Figure 7-13. Dissection between the right superior pulmonary vein and the inferior pulmonary vein.

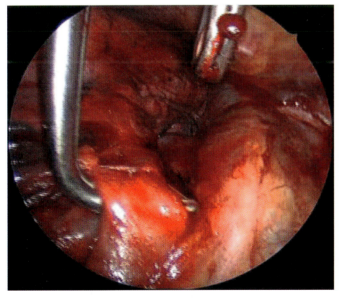

Figure 7-14. Right-angle clamp around the right superior pulmonary vein.

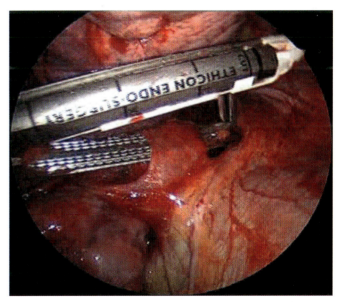

Figure 7-15. Stapler across the right superior pulmonary vein.

Step 3. Right Inferior Pulmonary Vein

◆ **Exposure:** Retract the lung directly toward the apex of the chest.
◆ Aim the thoracoscope anteriorly with the 30-degree lens pointed posteriorly.
◆ Retract the diaphragm with the curve of the Yankauer suction and with the tip of the suction pointed toward the inferior pulmonary ligament.
◆ A ring forceps through incision 3 retracts the lung directly toward the apex of the chest.
◆ The extension of the electrocautery through incision 1 takes down the inferior pulmonary ligament.
◆ Remove level 9 and 8 nodes with electrocautery.
◆ Retract the lung slightly posteriorly to dissect bluntly between the IPV and the SPV. This can be accomplished quickly with the Yankauer suction tip. The vein from the superior segment can be seen.
◆ Retract the lung anteriorly. Metzenbaum scissors through incision 1 incise the pleura posterior to the IPV. Dissection continues along the pericardium. A lymph node located posteriorly and superiorly to the IPV can be held with a ring forceps from incision 4. Removal of the node greatly facilitates IPV mobilization (Figure 7-16).
◆ Metzenbaum scissors, the Yankauer suction tip, or a right-angle clamp introduced through incision 1 or 3 passes around the IPV (Figure 7-17).
◆ A stapler through incision 1 or 3 transects the IPV.

Step 4. Right Subcarinal Node Dissection

◆ **Exposure:** Retract the lung directly anteriorly.
◆ Aim the thoracoscope anteriorly with the 30-degree lens pointed posteriorly.
◆ Retract the lung directly anteriorly with ring forceps.
◆ Metzenbaum scissors through incision 1 cut the pleura from the IPV to almost the level of the azygous vein.
◆ Blunt dissection with the Yankauer suction tip or the Metzenbaum scissors through incision 1 begins on the surface of the pericardium (Figure 7-18). A ring forceps from incision 4 holds the soft tissue in the subcarinal space. The esophagus and the vagus nerve constitute the posterior border for the dissection. There is a tendency to dissect toward the esophagus, but the dissection should be away from the esophagus and toward the bronchus.
◆ Using a ring forceps from incision 4, retract the esophagus posteriorly. This exposes the subcarinal nodes. When they are completely removed, the right and left mainstem bronchi are seen clearly (Figure 7-19).

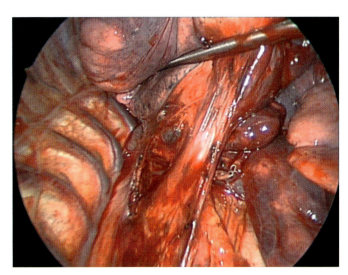

Figure 7-16. Posterior hilar node on the posterosuperior aspect of the right inferior pulmonary vein.

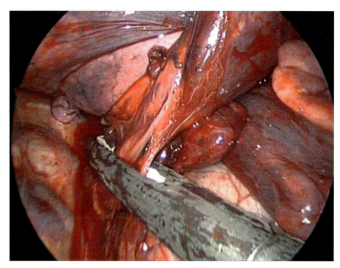

Figure 7-17. Stapling the right inferior pulmonary vein.

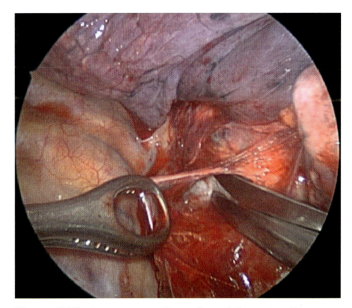

Figure 7-18. Dissection on the surface of the pericardium to start the subcarinal node dissection.

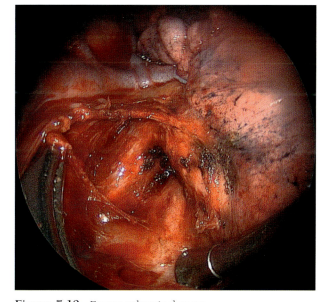

Figure 7-19. Empty subcarinal space.

Step 5. Right Pulmonary Artery

- **Exposure:** Retract the lung posteriorly and slightly inferiorly.
- Aim the thoracoscope anteriorly with the 30-degree lens pointed posteriorly.
- Blunt dissection with a Yankauer suction tip or Metzenbaum scissors through incision 3 separates the intermediate bronchus from the pericardium.
- The superior aspect of the right main pulmonary artery is well exposed after the level 10 nodes have been dissected. Blunt dissection with a Yankauer suction tip or Metzenbaum scissors through incision 3 mobilizes the inferior aspect of the artery away from the bronchus (Figure 7-20).
- Through incision 3, a right-angle clamp passes around the pulmonary artery after the blunt dissection has nearly completely mobilized the artery (Figure 7-21).
- Use an open stapler, such as the Covidien TA 30 or Ethicon TX 30 for the artery (Figure 7-22).

Step 6. Right Mainstem Bronchus

- **Exposure:** Retract the lung posteriorly and slightly inferiorly.
- Aim the thoracoscope anteriorly with the 30-degree lens pointed posteriorly.
- At this point, the right main bronchus is completely mobilized.
- Use an open stapler, such as the Covidien TA 30 or Ethicon TX 30 for the bronchus. Put the pin down, and pull the lung through the stapler to position the stapler as close as possible to the carina (Figure 7-23).
- Cut the bronchus with the Metzenbaum scissors or a scalpel through incision 3.

Step 7. Lung Removal

- **Exposure:** Retract the lung posteriorly and slightly inferiorly.
- Aim the thoracoscope posteriorly with the 30-degree lens pointed apically.
- Pull the lung with a ring forceps to the bottom of the chest to create a space for the removal bag.
- Using a ring forceps through incision 3, place the base of the Lapsac bag at the apex of the chest.
- With two ring forceps through incision 3, hold the bag open.
- Using a ring forceps from incision 4 or 1, push the lung into the bag. This usually takes several steps. When the lung is partially placed in the bag, the ring forceps pinches the lung, and the ring forceps that was holding the lung grabs a lower purchase on the lung and again pushes it into the bag.

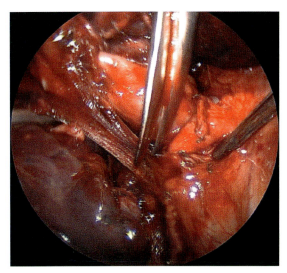

Figure 7-20. Dissection off the inferior aspect of the right main pulmonary artery.

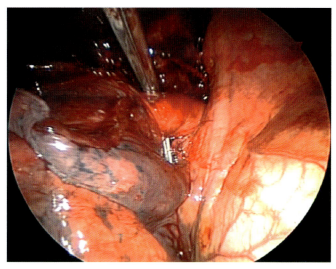

Figure 7-21. Right-angle clamp around the right main pulmonary artery.

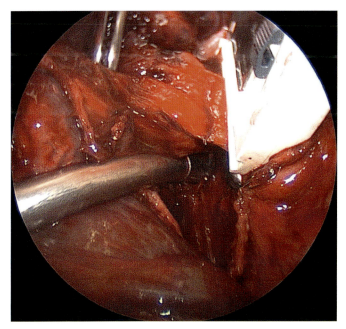

Figure 7-22. Stapler across the right main pulmonary artery.

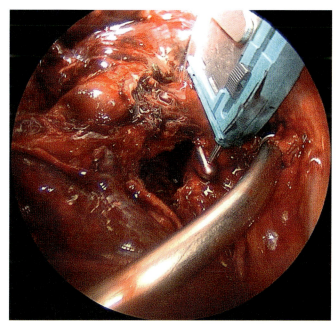

Figure 7-23. Stapler across the right mainstem bronchus.

CHAPTER 8

RIGHT UPPER LOBECTOMY — VIDEO 8

Robert J. McKenna, Jr.

Introduction

Right upper lobectomy can be performed as video-assisted thoracic surgery (VATS). Because the anatomy for the right upper lobe (RUL) is consistent, the approach to a lobectomy is straightforward.

Approach to Video-Assisted Right Upper Lobectomy

Order of Operative Steps

The order of the steps of the operation is as follows: level 10 nodes, RUL vein, anterior trunk of the pulmonary artery, minor fissure, posterior ascending artery, RUL bronchus, and the remainder of the fissure. The incisions are the standard incisions, with the utility incision placed directly up (lateral) from the superior pulmonary vein (see Chapter 1).

Key Points

- Work anteriorly to posteriorly with little manipulation of the lung.
- No posterior dissection is necessary.
- Complete resection of the tissue with the level 10 nodes exposes the right mainstem bronchus, superior vena cava (SVC), and anterior trunk. During dissection, the superior and posterior aspects of the anterior arterial trunk should be dissected well to mobilize the artery for subsequent transection.

 ### Video-Assisted Right Upper Lobectomy (Video 8-1)

Step 1. Level 10 Nodes

- **Exposure:** Retract lung posteriorly and slightly inferiorly.
- Aim the thoracoscope anteriorly with the 30-degree lens pointed posteriorly.
- The level 10 nodes are located within a triangle bounded by the SVC, azygous vein, and superior hilum of the lung.
- Just posterior and parallel to the phrenic nerve, incise the pleura from the hilum to the azygous vein and then posteriorly along the azygous vein to the right mainstem bronchus (Figure 8-1).
- From the hilum, dissect posteriorly along the superior aspect of the RUL vein and along the vein from the apical segment. This exposes the anterior trunk.

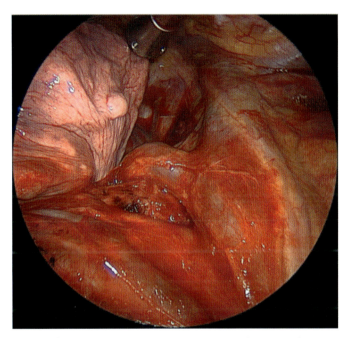

Figure 8-1. Level 10 nodes are removed by dissecting the triangle formed by the superior vena cava, the azygous vein, and the vein from the apex of the right upper lobe.

- Remove all the tissue in this triangle, including the level 10 nodes. At this point, the right mainstem bronchus, anterior trunk, and SVC are well exposed.
- After the level 10 nodes are removed, dissect along the superior aspect of the anterior trunk and posteriorly between the trunk and the right mainstem bronchus. This facilitates subsequent mobilization of the artery for later transection.

Step 2. Right Upper Lobe Vein

- **Exposure:** Retract the lung directly posteriorly.
- Aim the thoracoscope anteriorly with the 30-degree lens pointed posteriorly.
- Clearly identify the RUL vein and the right middle lobe vein. Viewing the remnant of the minor fissure can help with orientation.
- Spread along the inferior aspect of the RUL vein. Lifting the vein shows the plane between the vein and the underlying pulmonary artery.
- Rotate the thoracoscope posteriorly with the lens pointed anteriorly to view the dissection between the vein and the artery.
- Dissect along the superior aspect of the RUL vein.
- To create a tunnel for the stapler, spread widely with a right-angle clamp between the RUL vein and the artery (Figure 8-2).
- Through incision 4, pass an endoscopic vascular stapler around the RUL vein. The anvil goes into the tunnel between the vein and artery. The stapler can be passed through incision 1, but the angle is better from the posterior incision (Figure 8-3).

Step 3. Minor Fissure

- **Exposure:** Retract the lung inferiorly and directed toward the thoracoscope.
- The thoracoscope is aimed anteriorly with the 30-degree lens pointed posteriorly, but it is pulled back as close as possible to the trocar.
- Look at the minor fissure on the lateral surface of the lung and at the confluence of the RUL and right middle lobe veins to determine the exact location of the minor fissure.
- Point the anvil of the stapler toward this venous confluence, and hold it in place. Pull the lung parenchyma into the jaws of the endoscopic stapler without moving the stapler. This is a key maneuver and ensures that the stapler remains above all vascular structures and avoids inadvertent injury. The 4.8-mm staple cartridge typically is used for stapling lung parenchyma.
- The first firing of the stapler usually completes about one half of the fissure. Another stapler is positioned with the anvil of the stapler between the veins and on the surface of the artery (Figure 8-4).
- Open the jaws of the stapler, and with ring forceps, pull the lung parenchyma into the jaws of the stapler.
- Firing the stapler completes the minor fissure (Figure 8-5).

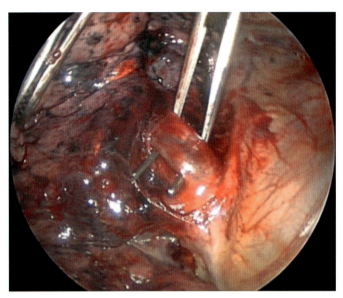

Figure 8-2. A right-angle instrument is passed around the right upper lobe vein, exposing the artery behind the vein.

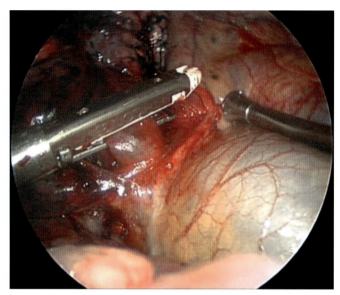

Figure 8-3. The stapler crosses the right upper lobe vein.

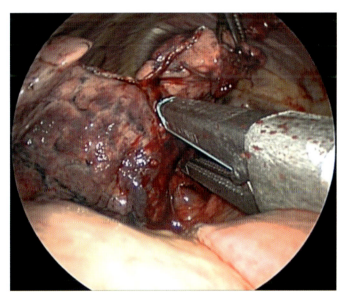

Figure 8-4. The anvil of the stapler is on the pulmonary artery in preparation for completing the minor fissure.

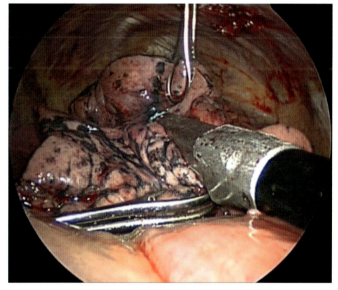

Figure 8-5. The stapler is not moved as the ring forceps pulls the lung parenchyma into the jaws of the stapler.

Step 4. Anterior Trunk

- **Exposure:** Retract the lung posteriorly and slightly inferiorly.
- The thoracoscope is positioned anteriorly with the 30-degree lens pointed posteriorly. Rotate the camera slightly clockwise.
- Sharply dissect the inferior aspect of the anterior trunk for 1 to 2 cm.
- Dissect the main right pulmonary artery to the level of the posterior ascending artery.
- Remove the lobar nodes between the anterior trunk and the main pulmonary artery.
- Mobilize the artery from the bronchus; a right-angle clamp then easily passes around the anterior trunk (Figure 8-6).
- With a stapler introduced from incision 4 (preferred) or incision 1, transect the artery (Figure 8-7).

Step 5. Define Right Upper Lobe Bronchus

- **Exposure:** Retract the lung directly posteriorly.
- The thoracoscope is aimed anteriorly with the 30-degree lens pointed posteriorly.
- Remove the lobar nodes that hide the surface of the RUL bronchus (Figure 8-8).
- Cauterize or clip the one or two small bronchial arteries to the bronchus and nodes.
- The posterior ascending artery can be seen inferiorly on the inferior border of the RUL bronchus.
- With Metzenbaum scissors, spread between the artery and the RUL bronchus until the vertebral bodies can be felt posteriorly (Figure 8-9). Be careful to not close the scissors when dissecting along the bronchus because that can cut the posterior ascending artery.

Step 6. Posterior Ascending Artery

- **Exposure:** Retract the lung directly posteriorly.
- The thoracoscope is aimed anteriorly with the 30-degree lens pointed posteriorly.
- With the lobar nodes on the RUL bronchus removed, the RUL bronchus and the posterior ascending artery can be seen clearly.
- Dissect bluntly along the posterior ascending artery to determine if there is a common trunk for that artery and the artery for the superior segment of the lower lobe.
- After the anatomy is clarified, double clip the origin of the posterior ascending artery (Figure 8-10). Do not clip the distal side of the artery because the clip would be in the staple line when the remainder of the fissure is stapled.
- The posterior ascending artery can then be cut distal to the two clips. This causes minor back bleeding, which can be ignored or the artery can be transected with the stapler that completes the posterior aspect of the fissure.

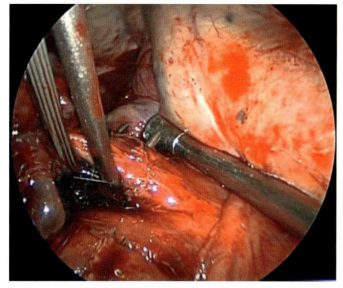

Figure 8-6. The right-angle clamp passes behind the anterior trunk.

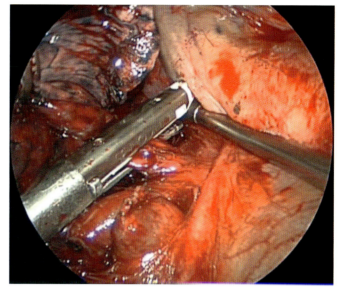

Figure 8-7. The stapler lies across the anterior trunk.

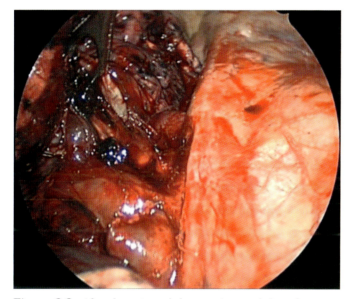

Figure 8-8. After the vein and the anterior trunk have been transected, the lymph nodes around the right upper lobe bronchus can be seen.

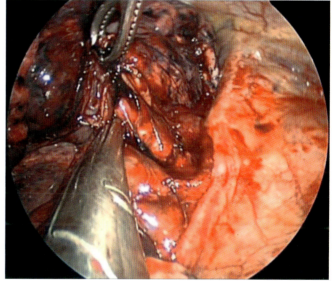

Figure 8-9. Through incision 1, the Metzenbaum scissors dissect along the inferior border of the right upper lobe bronchus.

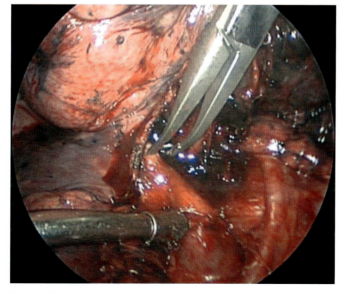

Figure 8-10. A clip is applied to the posterior ascending artery.

Step 7. Right Upper Lobe Bronchus

* **Exposure:** Retract the lung directly posteriorly.
* The thoracoscope is aimed anteriorly with the 30-degree lens pointed posteriorly.
* Spread the Metzenbaum scissors widely between the RUL bronchus and the posterior ascending artery. Remove the scissors before closing them, because they can cut the artery if they are closed before removal.
* Pass the endoscopic 4.8-mm stapler through incision 1. The anvil of the stapler is placed in the tunnel created by the scissors along the inferior border of the RUL bronchus. Fire the stapler (Figure 8-11).

Step 8. Completion of the Fissure

* **Exposure:** Retract the lung posteriorly and superiorly.
* The thoracoscope is aimed anteriorly with the 30-degree lens pointed posteriorly.
* Fire the endoscopic 4.8-mm stapler as many times as needed to complete the fissure (Figure 8-12).

Step 9. Lobe Removal

* **Exposure:** With a ring forceps through incision 4, hold the right lower lobe by the diaphragm to keep it out of view.
* The thoracoscope is aimed anteriorly with the 30-degree lens pointed to the apex of the chest for a panoramic view of the chest.
* With a ring forceps through the incision in the auscultatory triangle, the RUL is held posteriorly by the diaphragm to keep it out of view.
* Pass the Lapsac bag through the utility incision, push the base of the bag to the apex of the chest. With a ring forceps through the utility incision and another through the mid-clavicular incision, hold the bag widely open so the lobe can be inserted (Figure 8-13A).
* After the lobe is partially inserted into the bag, pinch the two ring forceps to hold the lobe in the bag (Figure 8-13B).
* With the ring through the auscultatory triangle, grasp a part of the lobe that is not in the bag, and push the remainder of the lobe into the bag.

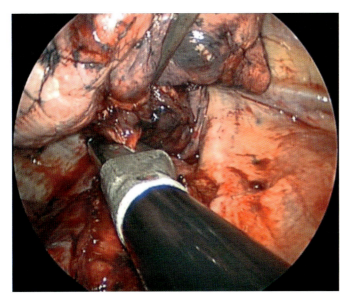

Figure 8-11. The stapler is positioned across the right upper lobe bronchus.

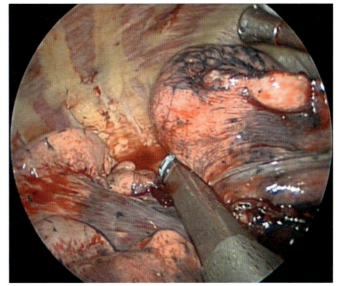

Figure 8-12. The stapler completes the fissure between the posterior segment of the right upper lobe and the superior segment of the right lower lobe.

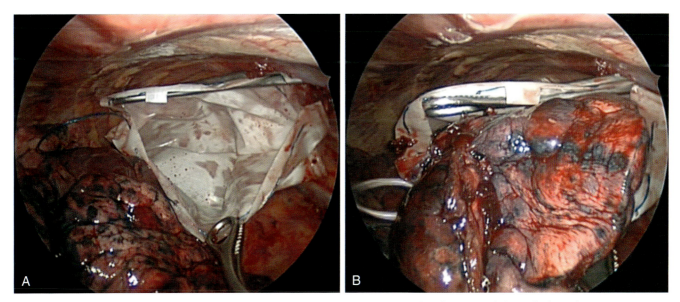

Figure 8-13. A, The bag is held open. **B,** The right upper lobe is placed into a bag for removal through the utility incision.

CHAPTER 9

RIGHT MIDDLE LOBECTOMY—VIDEO 9

Robert J. McKenna, Jr.

Introduction

The anatomic variations of the right middle lobe (RML) include an accessory artery posterior and inferior to the bronchus and the dual venous drainage to the superior pulmonary vein and the inferior pulmonary vein. The surgeon should be aware of these anatomic variations, but they have little impact on the operation.

Approach to Video-Assisted Right Middle Lobectomy

Order of Operative Steps

The order of steps for the operation is as follows: RML vein, major fissure between the RML and the right lower lobe (RLL), RML bronchus, RML artery, and the minor fissure. The incisions are described in Chapter 1 (see Figure 1-2). For a right middle lobectomy, place the utility incision (i.e., incision 3) one intercostal space below the superior pulmonary vein.

Key Points

- Work anteriorly to posteriorly with little manipulation of the lung.
- Approximately 20% of patients have an accessory middle lobe artery located inferior and posterior to the RML bronchus.
- Five percent of RMLs drain to the superior and inferior pulmonary veins.

Video-Assisted Right Middle Lobectomy

Step 1. Right Middle Lobe Vein

- **Exposure:** Retract the lung directly posteriorly.
- Aim the thoracoscope anteriorly with the 30-degree lens pointed posteriorly toward the hilum.
- Use the standard incisions, although the auscultatory incision is often not necessary (Figure 9-1). The utility incision is made directly up from the superior pulmonary vein, as for an upper lobectomy.
- Dissect between the inferior and superior pulmonary veins to define the inferior border of the RML vein, and determine whether there is drainage from the middle lobe to the inferior pulmonary vein.
- With DeBakey pickups and Metzenbaum scissors, define the superior and inferior aspect of the RML vein (Figure 9-2).
- Using the same exposure, dissect out the RML vein.
- Pass a right-angle clamp through the utility incision around the RML vein (Figure 9-3).
- With a vascular stapler from the utility incision or the auscultatory triangle incision, if used, transect the RML vein.

Step 2. Major Fissure

- **Exposure:** To line up the major fissure for stapling, retract the RLL inferiorly and slightly anteriorly while the RML is retracted inferiorly and medially to line up the major fissure with incision 1.
- Aim the thoracoscope anteriorly with the 30-degree lens pointed posteriorly and superiorly, directly down the fissure.
- Through incision 1, the anvil of the stapler is placed between the superior pulmonary vein and the inferior pulmonary vein. Hold the stapler in place as the lung parenchyma is pulled into the stapler. The cartridge of the stapler is lined up with the fissure, and the stapler is fired (Figure 9-4).
- Lift the remaining fissure with a ring forceps to expose the pulmonary artery in the fissure.
- Remove the lymph node between the RLL and RML bronchi.
- Define the pulmonary artery with the Metzenbaum scissors through incision 1 by spreading on the surface of the artery or with the Yankauer suction bluntly dissecting along the surface of the pulmonary artery.
- This dissection creates a tunnel for the stapler through incision 1 to complete the remainder of the major fissure to the level of the minor fissure.

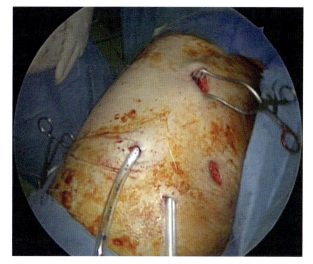

Figure 9-1. Standard incisions.

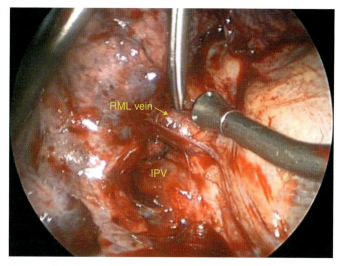

Figure 9-2. Dissection of the middle lobe vein.

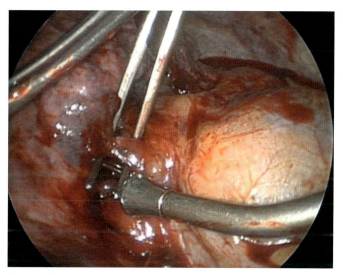

Figure 9-3. The inferior pulmonary vein and a right-angle clamp passing behind the right middle lobe vein.

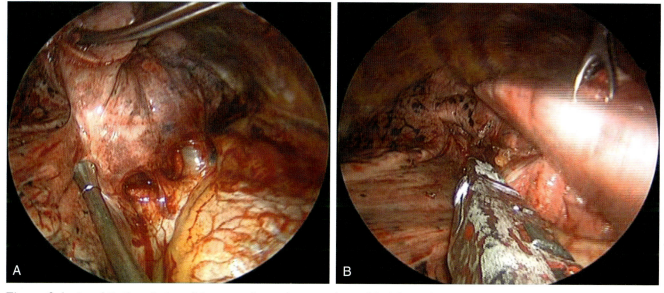

Figure 9-4. **A** and **B,** Completion of the major fissure between the middle lobe and the lower lobe.

Step 3. Accessory Right Middle Lobe Artery

- **Exposure:** Retract the RLL inferiorly and posteriorly, while the RML is retracted superiorly.
- Aim the thoracoscope anteriorly with the 30-degree lens pointed posteriorly.
- A few patients have an accessory right middle lobe artery that is located inferior and posterior to the RML bronchus (Figure 9-5).
- With DeBakey pickups and Metzenbaum scissors, dissect the artery away from the bronchus.
- A right-angle clamp introduced through the utility incision mobilizes the artery. The artery is usually small, and it can be clipped or tied.

Step 4. Right Middle Lobe Bronchus

- **Exposure:** Retract the RML toward the apex of the chest.
- Aim the thoracoscope anteriorly with the 30-degree lens pointed posteriorly but pulled back into the trocar.
- Remove the lobar nodes around the bronchus. Watch for the right middle lobe artery, which lies behind and parallel to the RML bronchus (Figure 9-6).
- With DeBakey pickups and Metzenbaum scissors introduced through the utility incision, dissect the bronchus away from the artery.
- Pass a right-angle clamp between the bronchus and the artery. Spread widely to create a tunnel for the stapler (Figure 9-7).
- Transect the bronchus with a stapler through the auscultatory or utility incision (Figure 9-8).

Step 5. Right Middle Lobe Artery

- **Exposure:** Retract the RLL posteriorly and inferiorly as the RML is retracted superiorly and anteriorly toward the apex of the chest.
- Aim the thoracoscope anteriorly with the 30-degree lens pointed posteriorly. The camera is rotated slightly clockwise.
- With the vein and bronchus transected, the RML artery is exposed as shown in Figure 9-9. Handling for the artery parallels that for the bronchus.
- With DeBakey pickups and Metzenbaum scissors introduced through the utility incision, dissect the artery. A right-angle clamp mobilizes the artery to create a tunnel through which the stapler will pass to transect the artery.
- Through the utility incision, a clip can be placed on the artery. Alternatively, a stapler (usually through the posterior incision) can transect the artery, or it can be tied.

Step 6. Minor Fissure

- **Exposure:** Retract the RLL posteriorly and inferiorly. A ring forceps through the midclavicular incision retracts the RML inferiorly.
- Aim the thoracoscope anteriorly with the 30-degree lens pointed posteriorly.
- Complete the minor fissure with a stapler that is brought through the utility incision.
- Place the anvil just inferior to the right upper lobe vein and on the surface of the artery (Figure 9-10).
- Line up the cartridge of the stapler with the minor fissure on the lateral surface of the lung. Hold the stapler stable as a ring forceps pulls the RML parenchyma into the stapler.
- Fire the stapler.

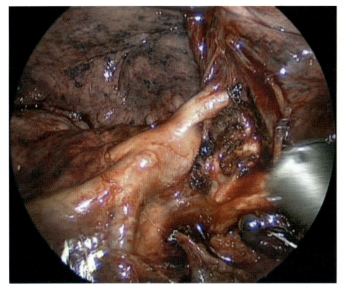

Figure 9-5. Accessory artery to the right middle lobe.

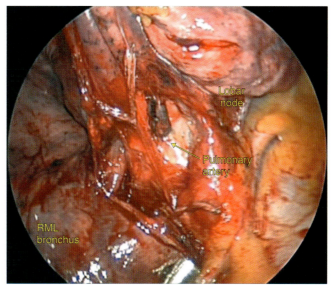

Figure 9-6. Relationships of the right middle lobe bronchus, right middle lobe artery, main pulmonary artery, and a lobar lymph node.

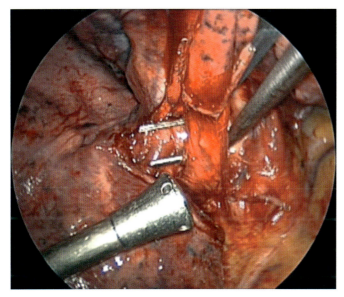

Figure 9-7. Right-angle clamp between the right middle lobe bronchus and the pulmonary artery.

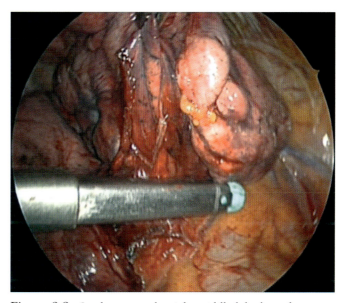

Figure 9-8. Stapler across the right middle lobe bronchus.

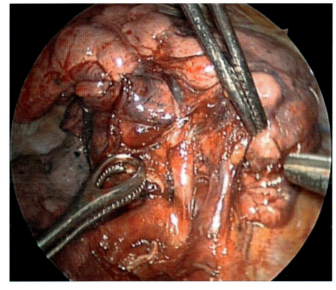

Figure 9-9. Relationships of the right middle lobe artery, right upper lobe vein, and pulmonary artery.

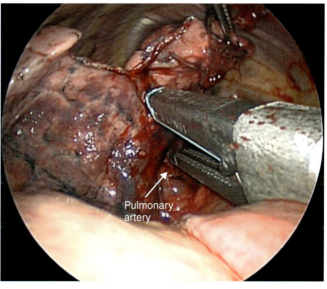

Figure 9-10. The anvil of the stapler is positioned on the pulmonary artery, inferior to the right upper lobe vein.

Step 7. Removal of the Lobe

+ **Exposure:** Retract the RML low in the chest near the diaphragm through the posterior auscultatory triangle incision.
+ Aim the thoracoscope anteriorly with the 30-degree lens pointed toward the apex of the chest for a panoramic view of the chest.
+ With a ring forceps through the incision in the auscultatory triangle, hold the RML posteriorly and inferiorly by the diaphragm to keep it out of view while the Lapsac bag is passed through the utility incision to the apex of the chest.
+ With a ring forceps through the utility incision and another through the mid-clavicular incision, hold the bag open so the lobe can be inserted.
+ Place the RML into the bag through the auscultatory triangle incision.
+ Through the utility incision, pull the bag out of the chest.

CHAPTER 10

RIGHT LOWER LOBECTOMY

Allan Pickens

Introduction

The bronchial and vascular anatomy of the right lower lobe is consistent, but the level at which these structures branch can vary. Proximal branching may require an alternate approach, and completeness of the fissure between adjacent lobes can greatly influence the surgical approach. The inferior and superior approaches to right lower lobectomy performed as video-assisted thoracic surgery (VATS) are described. The inferior approach involves isolating and transecting the lobar structures from an inferior to superior orientation. Sequentially, the vein, bronchus, and artery to the right lower lobe are transected. This approach reduces dissection in the fissure, which reduces the incidence of postoperative air leak. The superior approach transects the artery, vein, and bronchus. The superior approach is easier when the fissure is complete.

Approach to Video-Assisted Right Lower Lobectomy

Order of Operative Steps

The order of the steps of the operation is as follows: inferior pulmonary ligament takedown, inferior pulmonary vein ligation, right lower lobe bronchus ligation, right lower lobe pulmonary artery ligation, and major fissure completion for the inferior approach. The pulmonary artery is transected first when using the superior approach.

Key Points

- The utility incision is placed one intercostal space lower than the standard superior pulmonary vein level to allow better access to the structures in the lower thoracic cavity.
- Takedown of the inferior pulmonary ligament makes the lower lobe more mobile for palpation.
- The inferior approach avoids fissure dissection and potential air leaks when there is an incomplete fissure.
- The superior approach provides early arterial control when there is a complete fissure.
- Dissect close to the bronchus to avoid injuring the adjacent pulmonary artery.
- Do not compromise the right middle lobe vessels or bronchi when stapling lower lobe structures.
- Reinflation before stapling the bronchus can prevent compromise of the remaining airway.

Video-Assisted Right Lower Lobectomy

Step 1. Inferior Pulmonary Ligament Takedown
- **Exposure:** Retract the right lower lobe superiorly through the utility incision.
- The thoracoscope is aimed anteriorly with the 30-degree lens pointed posteriorly.
- Use electrocautery with an extended tip (or other energy source) to transect the inferior pulmonary ligament (Figure 10-1).
- Collect any station 9 inferior pulmonary ligament lymph nodes, and send them to pathology. Lymph nodes should be removed through the utility incision to avoid tumor implantation in smaller incisions.
- Electrocautery introduced from incision 1 transects the ligament up to the level of the right inferior pulmonary vein.
- Reposition the lung anteriorly, and continue to open the posterior hilar pleura. Remove the lymph nodes posterior and superior to the vein (Figure 10-2).

Step 2. Inferior Pulmonary Vein
- **Exposure:** The lung is retracted posteriorly and cephalad.
- The thoracoscope is aimed anteriorly with the 30-degree lens pointed posteriorly.
- Clearly identify the right inferior pulmonary vein. Ensure that the right middle lobe vein does not aberrantly drain into the right inferior pulmonary vein (Figure 10-3).

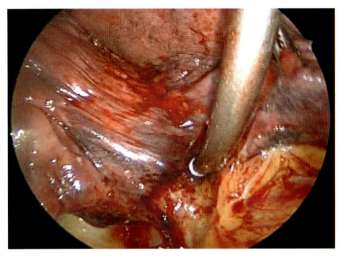

Figure 10-1. Suction dissects the superior aspect of the inferior pulmonary vein.

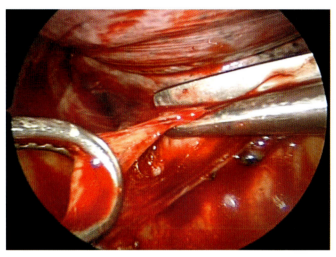

Figure 10-2. Dissection using Metzenbaum scissors directed posteriorly on the surface of the pericardium in preparation for removal of the subcarinal lymph nodes.

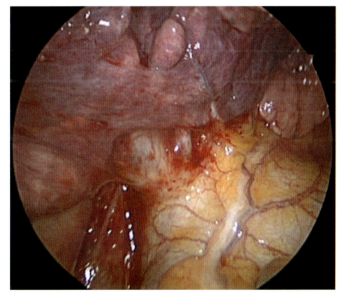

Figure 10-3. Aberrant drainage of the right middle lobe into the inferior pulmonary vein.

- Use Metzenbaum scissors and right-angle instruments to dissect along the superior border of the vein. Avoid injury to the back wall of the vein by directing instrument tips toward the bronchus (superiorly) rather than the vein wall.
- Introduce an endoscopic vascular stapler through the utility incision. A suture can be passed around the vessel for retraction if the stapler does not easily pass around the vessel.
- Pass the cartridge between the vein and the bronchus because it extends farther than the anvil (Figure 10-4); this approach ensures that the stapler completely crosses the vein before stapling (Figure 10-5). Have a sponge stick immediately available for tamponade if bleeding occurs. After transecting the vein, the RLL bronchus can be seen (Figure 10-6) and blunt dissection should prepare it for transection.
- With a Yankauer suction tip through incision 1, bluntly dissect on the inferior surface of the bronchus.

Step 3. Right Lower Lobe Pulmonary Artery

- **Exposure:** The lung is returned to its normal anatomic position.
- The thoracoscope is aimed anteriorly with the 30-degree lens pointed posteriorly. Intermittently, it is necessary to position the thoracoscope posteriorly with the 30-degree lens pointed anteriorly to see the opposite side of dissection.
- Metzenbaum scissors dissect on the surface of the artery (Figure 10-7) to create a tunnel for the stapler to complete the fissure. The right lower lobe pulmonary artery should be clearly visible. If not, gentle blunt dissection of the lung parenchyma can expose the vessel (Figure 10-8).
- Use Metzenbaum scissors or right-angle instruments to dissect the right lower lobe pulmonary artery away from the lung parenchyma. Remain on guard for pulmonary artery branches that may not be visible. Do not force instruments during dissection.
- Suture may be used to encircle and gently retract vessels for insertion of endoscopic vascular staplers.
- Avoid tension on the pulmonary artery during use of the stapler. Stabilize the stapler at the chest wall level to prevent movement during stapling (Figure 10-9).

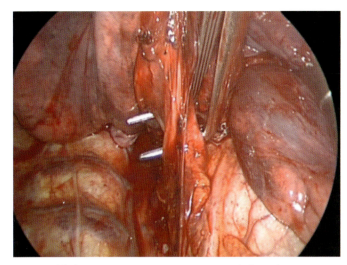

Figure 10-4. Right-angle instrument around the inferior pulmonary vein.

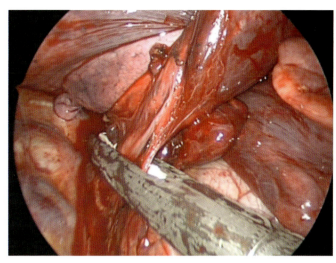

Figure 10-5. Stapler across the inferior pulmonary vein.

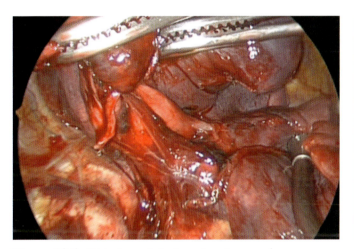

Figure 10-6. Right lower lobe bronchus is seen after transection of the vein.

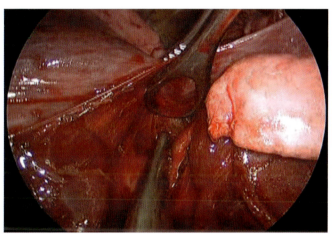

Figure 10-7. Scissors dissect on the surface of the artery to create a tunnel for the stapler to complete the fissure.

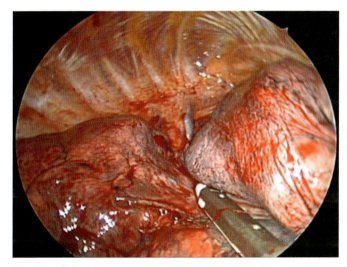

Figure 10-8. The stapler completes the fissure.

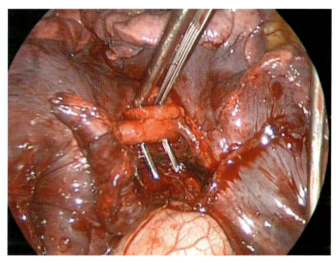

Figure 10-9. Right angle dissects the right lower lobe artery.

- Ensure that the vascular stapler completely crosses the artery before firing.
- Have a sponge stick readily available to tamponade the artery if bleeding occurs.
- Visualize the artery well to see that the stapler will not compromise a possible accessory artery for the right middle lobe, as seen in Figure 10-10.

Step 4. Right Lower Lobe Bronchus

- **Exposure:** The lung is in the normal anatomic position.
- The thoracoscope is aimed anteriorly with the 30-degree lens pointed posteriorly. Intermittently, it is necessary to position the thoracoscope posteriorly with the 30-degree lens pointed anteriorly to see the opposite side of dissection.
- Any lymph nodes that obstruct the view of the bronchus should be removed separately or swept so that they can be removed en bloc with the specimen.
- Use cautery (or other energy source) for any small bronchial vessels. Avoid clips because they can disrupt later stapling.
- Use Metzenbaum scissors or right-angle instruments to dissect the right lower lobe bronchus away from the underlying pulmonary artery. Avoid injury to the pulmonary artery by keeping instrument tips close to the bronchus.
- Create the dissection plane distal to the right middle lobe bronchus but proximal to the bronchus to the superior segment of the right lower lobe. If this is not possible because of the proximity of the bifurcation, dissect and transect the right lower lobe superior segment bronchus separately.
- Bring an endoscopic stapler for thick tissue (usually a green load cartridge) into the chest through the utility incision and across the bronchus (Figure 10-11). Close the stapler without firing. Reinflation of the lung at this time helps to ensure that the correct bronchus is occluded and that there is no impingement on other bronchi (i.e., right middle lobe bronchus). Ensure there are no devices within the airway, and fire the stapler (Figure 10-12). Alternatively, if the stapler is rotated counterclockwise, the middle lobe bronchus can be clearly seen to avoid compromising it with the staple (Figure 10-12).

Step 5. Major Fissure Completion

- **Exposure:** The lung is retracted laterally.
- The thoracoscope is aimed anteriorly with the 30-degree lens pointed posteriorly.
- Using a tissue stapler (usually a green load cartridge for thick tissue) placed through incision 1, complete the fissure (Figure 10-13).
- Pull lung parenchyma into the stapler for maximum efficiency.
- The lung parenchyma must be elevated laterally to expose the previously transected structures and avoid damaging staple lines.

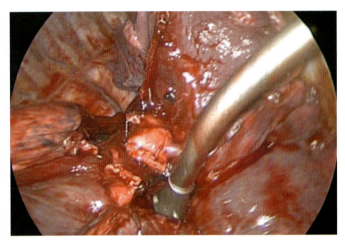

Figure 10-10. Transected artery of the right lower lobe shows preservation of the right middle lobe artery.

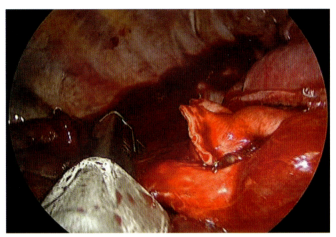

Figure 10-11. Stapler across the right lower lobe bronchus.

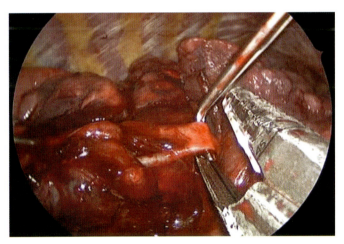

Figure 10-12. A right angle and stapler around the right lower lobe artery

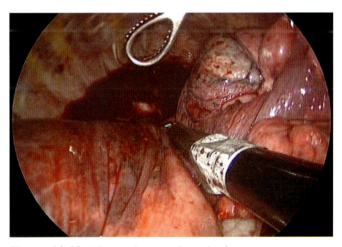

Figure 10-13. The stapler completes the fissure.

CHAPTER 11

LEFT UPPER LOBECTOMY—

VIDEO 11

Ali Mahtabifard

Introduction

The variability of the blood supply to the left upper lobe makes left upper lobectomy performed by video-assisted thoracic surgery (VATS) the most challenging minimally invasive lobectomy. This operation should be performed with the utmost care. There may be as many as seven arterial branches to the left upper lobe.

Approach to Video-Assisted Left Upper Lobectomy

Order of Operative Steps

The order of the steps for a left upper lobectomy is as follows: level 5 and 6 nodes, superior pulmonary vein (SPV), anterior trunk, fissure, lingular artery, bronchus, remaining arterial branches, and any remaining fissure.

Key Points

* Because isolation of the left upper lobe bronchus is a partially blind dissection between the bronchus and the artery, it is the most dangerous step. The main pulmonary artery (PA) resides posterior to the left upper lobe bronchus, and it can be damaged during the bronchial dissection.
* Removal of the level 5 and 6 lymph nodes and dissection along the superior aspect of the hilum mobilizes the superior and posterior aspects of the anterior trunk of the PA. This greatly facilitates the subsequent dissection of the anterior trunk.

 ## Video-Assisted Left Upper Lobectomy

Step 1: Incisions

* Incisions 1 and 2 can be moved slightly posteriorly to avoid the pericardium (see Chapter 5).
* The utility incision is located directly over the superior pulmonary vein for an upper lobectomy.
* If a diagnosis of lung cancer has not been made preoperatively, the utility incision is initially only 2 cm long for the wedge resection. When the diagnosis of cancer is made, this utility incision is lengthened to 4 to 5 cm for the lobectomy, and incision 4 is made.

Step 2: Resection of Level 5 and 6 Nodes

- **Exposure:** The lung is retracted posteriorly and slightly inferiorly with a ring forcep through the posterior incision.
- The thoracoscope is aimed anteriorly with the 30-degree lens pointed toward the hilum.
- Moving from the hilum to the aorta, incise the pleura just posterior to the phrenic nerve.
- Bring the Metzenbaum scissors through the inferior incision, and lift the hilar tissue with the long DeBakey forceps, which is brought through the utility incision.
- The scissors should be rotated so the tips of the scissors do not obstruct visualization of the phrenic nerve.
- Cut just the pleura, because cutting the vascular, underlying fat causes nuisance bleeding.
- Incise the pleura along the superior aspect of the vein draining the apex of the left upper lobe (LUL).
- Dissect on named structures.
- Use a combination of sharp and blunt dissection to dissect along the SPV and then the PA. Blunt dissection is often performed with the sucker tip.

Step 3: Superior Hilar Dissection

- **Exposure:** Retract the lung posteriorly and inferiorly through the posterior incision.
- Aim the thoracoscope slightly anteromedially and the lens slightly posteriorly.
- Dissection is carried cephalad along the edge of the SPV over the superior hilum.
- As the vein is mobilized, the anterior trunk is visualized.
- Dissection of the fat and level 5 lymph nodes away from the vessels greatly facilitates subsequent mobilization of the artery and vein for subsequent transection (Figure 11-1).

Step 4: Station 5 and 6 Lymph Node Dissection

- **Exposure:** Retract the lung posteriorly and inferiorly through the posterior incision.
- The thoracoscope is aimed anteriorly with the 30-degree lens pointed toward the mediastinum.
- Lift the anteroposterior lymph nodes with a ring forceps to dissect on the surface of the SPV and the PA. Identify the vagus and recurrent laryngeal nerves in this region, so they can be kept out of harm's way.
- Station 6 (para-aortic) lymph nodes are dissected away from the aorta and the pericardium. To achieve this, the retraction on the lung is not changed, but the 30-degree lens is pointed medially.
- The phrenic nerve is carefully elevated, not grasped. The station 6 lymph node packet can be grasped with ring forceps and bluntly dissected.
- Electrocautery should be used sparingly in this region to decrease the chance of nerve injury.
- Any minor bleeding can be controlled with Surgicel in this region.

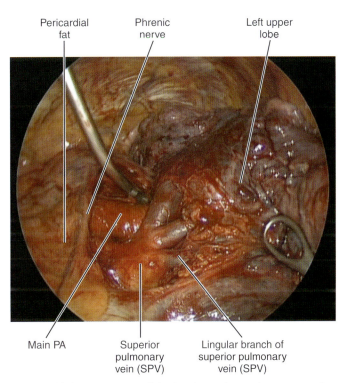

Figure 11-1. Dissection of the level 5 and 6 nodes exposes the superior aspect of the superior pulmonary vein.

Step 5: Superior Pulmonary Vein

- **Exposure:** The lung is retracted laterally and posteriorly through the posterior and anterior incisions.
- The thoracoscope is aimed anteriorly and slightly medially, and the lens is pointed toward the mediastinum and slightly posteriorly.
- Dissect the inferior border of the SPV. Bring the Metzenbaum scissors through the inferior incision while passing the Yankauer suction through the utility incision.
- Define the inferior pulmonary vein to ensure there is not a common trunk for the superior and inferior veins.
- A ring forceps through the utility incision lifts the entire SPV for the Metzenbaum scissors to dissect between the SPV and the LUL bronchus, which is just posterior to the SPV. A large purchase on the vein minimizes the chances of damaging the SPV, whereas a small purchase may tear the vessel.
- The vein is lifted as the Metzenbaum scissors dissects between the SPV and the LUL bronchus.
- After this dissection is complete, use the Metzenbaum scissors through the utility incision to complete dissection on the superior border of the SPV.
- Pass a right-angle clamp behind the SPV (Figure 11-2).
- A tie around the vein may elevate the vein to facilitate passing the stapler around the vein, although this is not often needed.
- A nonreticulating vascular stapler introduced through the posterior incision transects the vein (Figure 11-3).

Step 6: Anterior Trunk

- **Exposure:** The lung is retracted laterally and inferiorly through the posterior incision.
- The thoracoscope is aimed anteriorly, and the lens is pointed slightly posteriorly.
- After stapling the SPV, the anterior trunk of the PA is readily visualized. Incise the lymphatics on the superior aspect of the LUL bronchus, and remove lymph nodes to better expose the PA. Remove the lymph node between the bifurcation of the anterior trunk and the main PA for easier isolation of the anterior trunk (Figure 11-4).

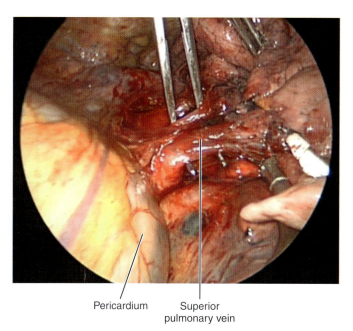

Pericardium   Superior
                pulmonary vein

Figure 11-2. A right-angle clamp is passed around the superior pulmonary vein.

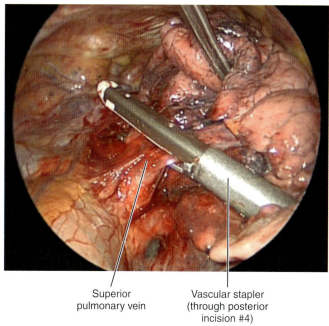

Superior   Vascular stapler
pulmonary vein   (through posterior
                    incision #4)

Figure 11-3. The stapler introduced from the posterior incision transects the superior pulmonary vein.

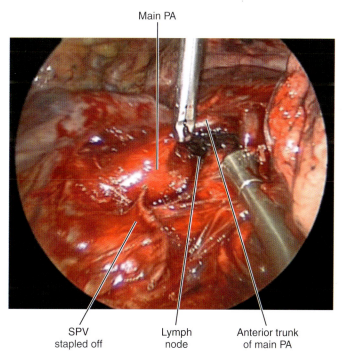

Main PA

SPV   Lymph   Anterior trunk
stapled off node   of main PA

Figure 11-4. The lobar node is removed between the takeoff of the anterior trunk and the main pulmonary artery (PA).

- A right-angle clamp introduced through the utility incision passes around the anterior trunk of the PA (Figure 11-5). Adjust the angle of the camera to allow complete visualization of the right-angle clamp as it encircles the anterior trunk. There should be little or no resistance to the passage of the right-angle clamp after prior dissection of the superior aspect of the hilum. The right-angle clamp is spread widely to create an adequate tunnel for subsequent stapler placement.
- The vascular stapler is brought through the posterior incision and placed across the anterior trunk. The anvil of the stapler should be placed in the tunnel between the PA and the anterior trunk (Figure 11-6).

Step 7: Fissure
- **Exposure:** The lung is returned to its anatomic position. Through the posterior incision, the lower lobe is retracted posteriorly, and through the utility incision, the upper lobe is retracted anteriorly.
- The thoracoscope is aimed anteriorly, and the 30-degree lens is pointed down the fissure.
- For an incomplete fissure, the stapler introduced through incision 1 separates the lingula from the lower lobe (Figure 11-7). The stapler is well away from the PA in patients with an incomplete fissure.

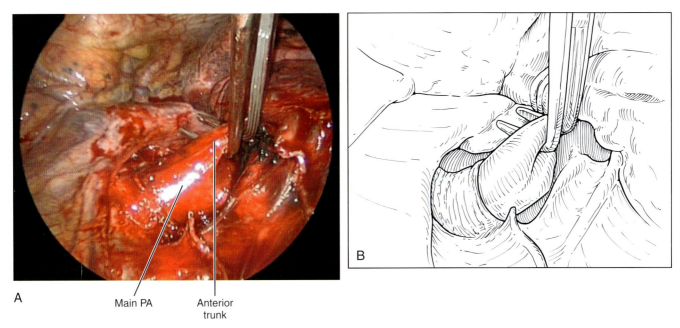

A

Main PA   Anterior
              trunk

B

Figure 11-5. **A** and **B,** A right-angle clamp is passed around the anterior trunk.

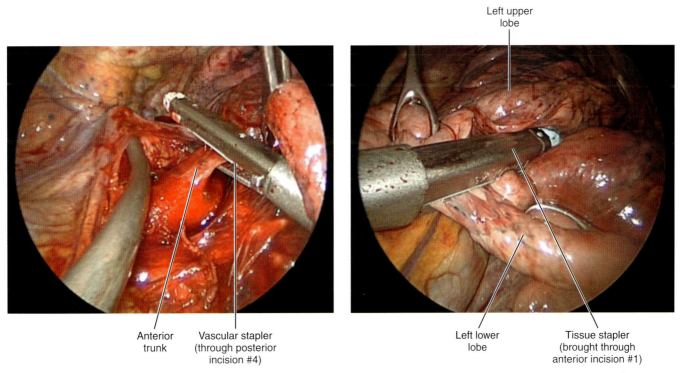

Left upper
lobe

Anterior   Vascular stapler
trunk   (through posterior
            incision #4)

Left lower   Tissue stapler
lobe   (brought through
              anterior incision #1)

Figure 11-6. The stapler introduced from the posterior incision transects the anterior trunk.

Figure 11-7. The stapler completes the anterior aspect of the fissure.

- To complete the remainder of the fissure, a tunnel is created on the surface of the PA.
- A ring forceps lifts the lung parenchyma of the incomplete fissure away from the surface of the artery (Figure 11-8).
- The LUL and the left lower lobe (LLL) bronchi are identified. A lymph node between the bronchi is removed to expose the PA, which runs parallel to and adjacent to the LLL bronchus.
- Use Metzenbaum scissors through incision 1 to dissect on the surface of the PA to create a tunnel. The dissection is on the anterior surface of the PA. On the superior side of the PA are the lingular and posterior ascending arteries, and on the inferior aspect of the PA is the artery to the superior segment of the LLL.
- When an adequate tunnel has been created on the surface of the artery, the stapler completes the fissure. The anvil of the stapler is placed into the tunnel and rests on the surface of the artery. *Once in position, the stapler is not moved. This is a key maneuver* (Figure 11-9).

Stump of
anterior trunk

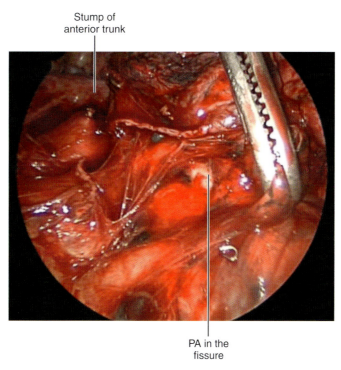

PA in the
fissure

Figure 11-8. Anterior exposure of the pulmonary artery.

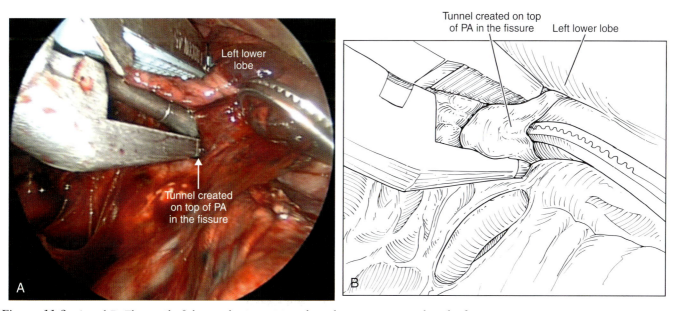

Figure 11-9. A and **B**, The anvil of the stapler is positioned on the artery to complete the fissure.

◆ While the stapler is held in position, ring forceps on the upper and lower lobes pull the lung parenchyma into the stapler. My colleagues and I typically use a 4.8-mm stapler to complete the fissure. However, if the fissure is well developed and there is not much lung parenchyma to be stapled, smaller (vascular) staples may be used.

◆ Repeat the process of opening the fissure by creating the tunnel until the fissure is completed. The PA and the bronchus should be clearly visualized.

◆ The left upper lobe bronchus, the main PA, and the lingular artery are readily identified (Figure 11-10).

Step 8: Lingular Artery

◆ **Exposure:** The exposure remains the same as in step 7.

◆ The camera angle remains the same as in step 7.

◆ Metzenbaum scissors brought through the inferior incision dissect the lingular artery. After adequate dissection is accomplished, the right-angle clamp is brought through the utility incision to mobilize the lingular artery by spreading widely enough to make room for the anvil of the stapler (Figure 11-11).

◆ The lingular artery can be stapled using the vascular stapler, which is brought through the inferior incision (Figure 11-12) or through the posterior incision.

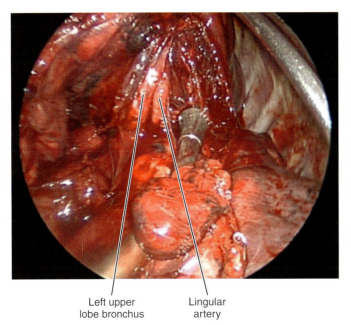

Left upper   Lingular
lobe bronchus   artery

Figure 11-10. Exposure of the bronchus and the lingular artery after the fissure has been opened.

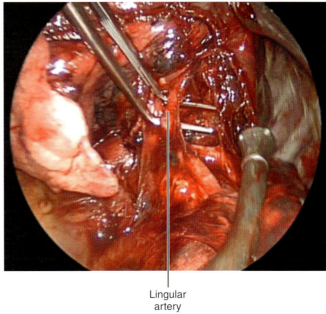

Lingular
artery

Figure 11-11. The right-angle clamp is passed around the lingular artery.

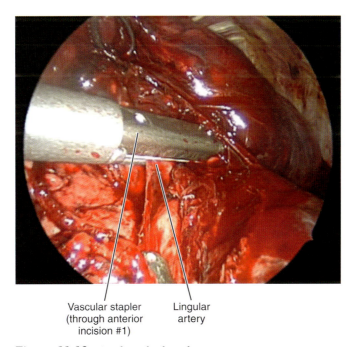

Vascular stapler   Lingular
(through anterior   artery
incision #1)

Figure 11-12. Stapling the lingular artery.

Step 9: Upper Lobe Bronchus

- **Exposure:** The exposure remains the same as in step 8.
- The camera angle remains the same as in step 8.
- Encircling and isolation of this bronchus is the most dangerous move in VAB left upper lobectomy, because it is partially a blind move between the bronchus and the main PA.
- Ring forceps through the utility incision lift the LUL bronchus away from the PA. Facilitate visualization of the posterior aspect of the bronchus by lifting it away from the PA. Aim the thoracoscope posteriorly, and point the lens anteriorly.
- Blunt dissection on the PA separates the bronchus and the PA.
- Use Metzenbaum scissors brought through the inferior incision to dissect the inferior border of the left upper lobe bronchus.
- Dissect the superior aspect of the LUL bronchus. Visualization of the superior aspect of the bronchus is achieved by retracting the bronchus posteriorly while the thoracoscope is pointed anteriorly and the lens is pointed posteriorly. Blunt dissection on the surface of the artery separates the bronchus from the PA.
- At this point, the bronchus is almost completely separated from the PA. The right-angle clamp is brought through the utility incision and is passed between the upper lobe bronchus and the PA (Figure 11-13).
- *This move is the only partially blind move in this operation and should be done with care to prevent damage to the PA, which resides just behind the bronchus.* Continuously manipulate the angle of the thoracoscope to enable maximal control and viewing of the right-angle clamp as it encircles the bronchus.
- Widely spread the right-angle clamp to create a tunnel for the stapler, which is introduced through the posterior incision to transect the bronchus (Figure 11-14).

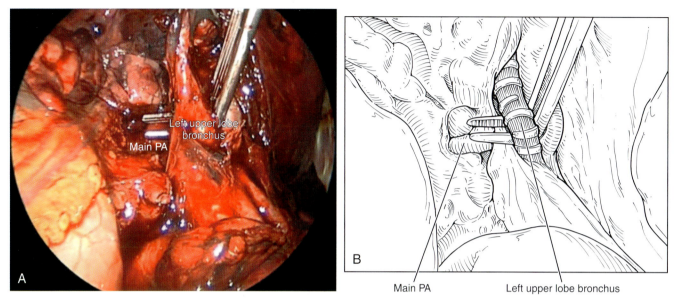

Figure 11-13. A and **B,** The right-angle clamp is passed around the left upper lobe bronchus.

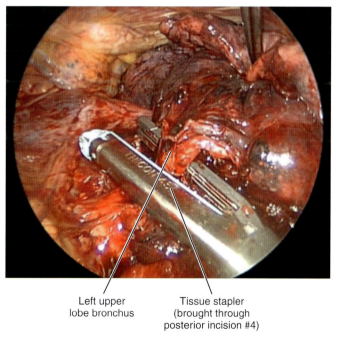

Figure 11-14. Stapling the left upper lobe bronchus.

Step 10: Remaining Arterial Branches

- **Exposure:** A ring clamp through the utility incision lifts the upper lobe to expose any remaining arterial branches to the left upper lobe.
- The thoracoscope is positioned with the 30-degree lens pointing medially, and the lens pointing posteriorly.
- Begin a combination of blunt and sharp dissection on the surface of the main PA to expose any remaining arterial branches to the left upper lobe.
- There may be up to five additional arterial branches that can be stapled, clipped, or tied (Figures 11-15 and 11-16).
- A 4.8-mm stapler through the inferior incision completes the remainder of the fissure (Figure 11-17).
- The disconnected lobe is brought down to the diaphragm and then placed inside the Lapsac as previously described in Chapter 7.

Left upper
lobe

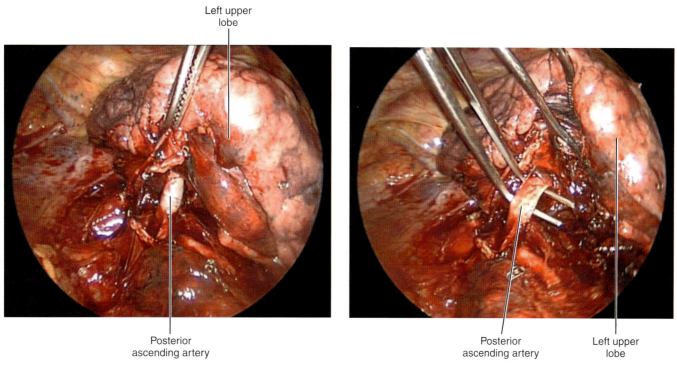

Posterior
ascending artery

Posterior
ascending artery

Left upper
lobe

Figure 11-15. Posterior ascending artery.

Figure 11-16. A right-angle clamp is used to mobilize the posterior ascending artery.

Left upper
lobe

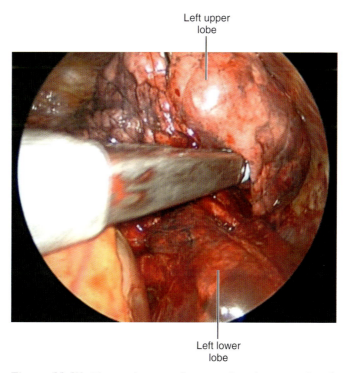

Left lower
lobe

Figure 11-17. The stapler is used to complete the remainder of the fissure.

CHAPTER 12

LEFT LOWER LOBECTOMY—
VIDEO 12

Ali Mahtabifard

Introduction

The preoperative care, indications, and patient positioning for left lower lobectomy are similar to those outlined in preceding chapters and are not repeated here.

Approach to Video-Assisted Left Lower Lobectomy

Order of Operative Steps

The order of the steps for a left lower lobectomy is as follows: inferior pulmonary vein (IPV), inferior aspect of the fissure, artery, bronchus, and remainder of the fissure.

Key Points

- The utility incision is placed one interspace lower than that for an upper lobectomy.
- Always dissect on named structures.
- Remove lymph nodes to define anatomy.
- Open the fissure to identify arterial branches.

Video-Assisted Left Lower Lobectomy

Step 1: Incisions

- Standard incisions are described in Chapter 1 (see Figure 1-2).

Step 2: Inferior Pulmonary Ligament and Level 9 Lymph Nodes

- **Exposure:** Retract the lung superiorly and slightly posteriorly through the utility incision.
- Aim the thoracoscope anteriorly, and point the 30-degree lens toward the inferior pulmonary ligament.

- Retract the lower lobe superiorly with a ring forceps through the utility incision. Apply enough tension to keep the inferior pulmonary ligament on stretch (Figure 12-1).
- Bring the cautery with an extension and the Yankauer suction into the chest through incision 1. If the diaphragm obstructs the view, push the diaphragm inferiorly with the Yankauer suction positioned so that its "bend" pushes the diaphragm downward while the tip is pointed toward the dissection to suck the smoke from the electrocautery.
- Remove the level 9 lymph nodes from within the inferior pulmonary ligament.
- Alternatively, if the diaphragm is high and obstructing the view, retract it downward with a stitch. A needle holder through incision 1 places a suture in the ligamentous portion of the diaphragm, near the esophageal hiatus. Bring the suture with its needle out through incision 2. Pull it as tightly as possible and suture it to the chest wall inferior to incision 2.
- Cauterize the inferior pulmonary ligament parallel to the esophagus up to the level of the inferior pulmonary vein (IPV) (Figure 12-2).

Step 3: Posterior Pleura
- **Exposure:** Retract the lung anteromedially and superiorly.
- Aim the thoracoscope posteriorly with the 30-degree lens pointed medially toward the heart.
- With the lung retracted anteromedially, open the posterior pleura along the posterior surface of the IPV. Use a combination of sharp dissection with the Metzenbaum scissors and the long-tipped electrocautery, which are brought through anterior incision (Figure 12-3).
- The line of dissection posteriorly should be at the junction of the pleura and the lung parenchyma.
- Dissection too close to the esophagus can cause unnecessary bleeding from its muscle fibers.
- In the course of this dissection, cut branches of the vagus nerve to the lung, and clip or cauterize bronchial arteries. Perform blunt dissection on the surface of the pericardium.
- Remove the lymph node on the posterosuperior aspect of the IPV. This is marked as a posterior hilar lymph node.

Step 4: Inferior Pulmonary Vein
- **Exposure:** Retract the lung posteriorly and superiorly to allow dissection of the hilum.
- Aim the thoracoscope medially with the 30-degree lens pointed posteriorly and laterally.
- The inferior border of the IPV should be well defined at this point (see step 2).
- With the Metzenbaum scissors brought through the anterior incision, cut the pleura at its junction with the pericardium. Define the superior aspect of the IPV, and perform blunt or sharp dissection between the IPV and the superior pulmonary vein (SPV), as shown in Figure 12-4. The vein from the superior segment can be seen.

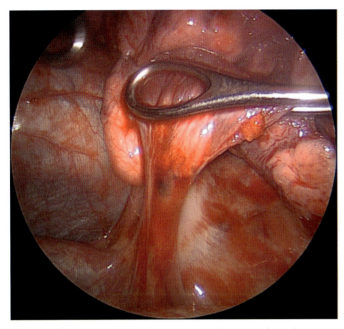

Figure 12-1. The lower lobe is retracted superiorly with a ring forceps through the utility incision. This maneuver places the inferior pulmonary ligament on stretch.

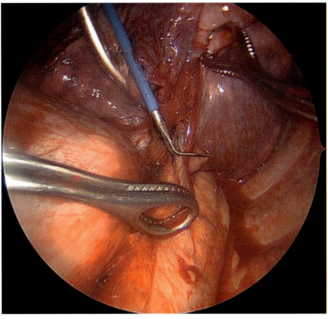

Figure 12-2. The inferior pulmonary ligament is cauterized through incision 1 up to the level of the inferior pulmonary vein. At this time, level 9 lymph nodes are excised.

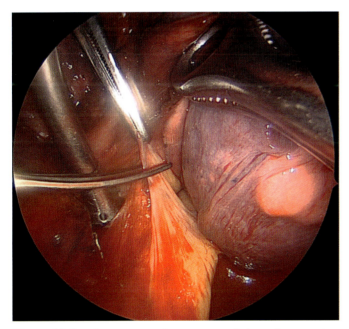

Figure 12-3. The posterior pleura is opened along the posterior surface of the inferior pulmonary vein. Dissection too close to the esophagus can cause bleeding from its muscle fibers.

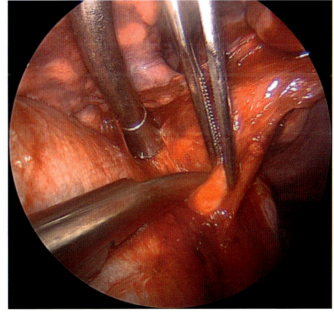

Figure 12-4. From the anterior aspect of the hilum, the superior aspect of the inferior pulmonary vein is defined. Sharp dissection is performed between the inferior pulmonary vein and the superior pulmonary vein. With repeated spreads, the Metzenbaum scissors will "fall through."

- Pass a right-angle clamp through the utility incision around the IPV. Because of the previously performed dissections on the anterior and posterior aspects of the IPV, the right-angle clamp should pass with little effort. Spread the right angle widely to create a tunnel for the stapler (Figure 12-5).
- Bring a vascular endoscopic stapler through the anterior or utility incision to staple the vein. If the staple cartridge is placed in the tunnel created by the right angle, it is easier to see that the stapler is completely across the vein (Figure 12-6).
- If the stapler is not completely across the entire vein, partial firing or misfiring of the stapler at this point can lead to massive, life-threatening hemorrhage.
- Keep a sponge stick readily available throughout this operation to control bleeding with direct pressure.
- After transecting the vein, the bronchus can be seen. Remove the lobar nodes from the bronchus, and perform blunt dissection with this exposure to prepare the bronchus for subsequent transection.

Step 5: Subcarinal Lymph Node Dissection

- **Exposure:** With a ring forceps through the utility incision and a long, curved ring forceps through the lower anterior incision, retract the lower lobe superiorly and medially.
- Aim the thoracoscope laterally with the 30-degree lens pointed medially.
- Dissection of the subcarinal lymph nodes is more difficult on the left than on the right. If it is done before the lower lobe has been removed, pulling on the lower lobe can help to open the space for the nodal dissection. With the previously described exposure, carry the dissection cephalad to the subcarinal space for the lymph node removal.
- The planes of dissection should be the pericardium medially and the esophagus posterolaterally. Dissect parallel but anterior to the esophagus and the vagus nerve. Dissecting too close to the esophagus can cause nuisance bleeding and possibly cause esophageal injury.
- Retract the esophagus posteriorly to open the subcarinal space. A ring forceps can be opened widely to open the subcarinal space for nodal dissection.
- After the subcarinal space is reached, lymph nodes can be taken out and sent to the pathology department as separate specimens. With thorough dissection, the carina and the right mainstem bronchus are visualized (Figure 12-7).
- Remove the subcarinal nodes through the utility incision to prevent seeding the smaller incisions with cancer cells.

Step 6: Completing the Fissure

- **Exposure:** Return the lung to its anatomic position. Grasp the lower lobe with a ring forceps through the posterior incision, and grasp the upper lobe with a ring forceps through the utility incision. Subsequent dissection and stapling is done through the anterior incision.
- Place the thoracoscope in a neutral position, and point the 30-degree lens posteriorly.
- If the fissure is not complete (as is often the case), fire a tissue stapler across the fissure to separate the lower lobe and the lingula (Figure 12-8). This initial firing is peripheral enough to be well away from the pulmonary artery. This advances the dissection into the fissure and closer to the bronchus and the artery.
- A lobar node between the upper and lower lobe bronchus hides the pulmonary artery; remove this lobar node to expose the artery.

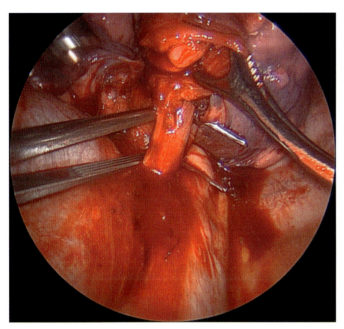

Figure 12-5. The right-angle clamp is brought through the utility incision and maneuvered around the inferior pulmonary vein. The right-angle clamp is spread widely to create a tunnel for the stapler.

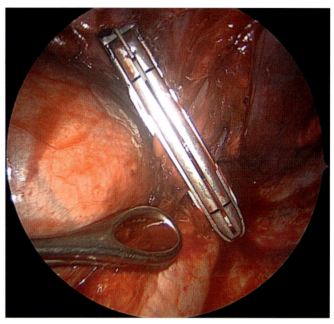

Figure 12-6. The inferior pulmonary vein is stapled from the utility incision. Alternatively, incision 1 can be used for the stapler. The cartridge is placed in the tunnel.

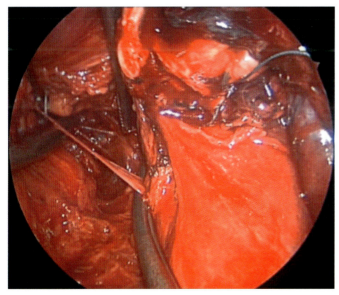

Figure 12-7. With thorough subcarinal dissection, the carina and the right mainstem bronchus can be visualized from the left side.

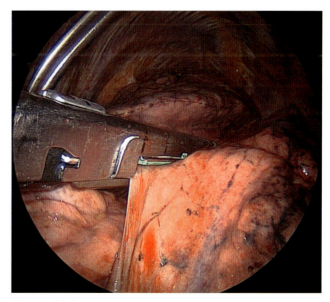

Figure 12-8. Peripherally, a tissue stapler across the fissure separates the lower lobe and the lingular segment of the left upper lobe.

- To complete the remainder of the fissure, create a tunnel on the surface of the artery with blunt dissection or sharp dissection with the Metzenbaum scissors through incision 1 (Figure 12-9).
- Expose the artery by lifting the lung parenchyma with ring forceps and working on the *surface of the artery*. Take care not to injure the artery.
- Place the anvil of the stapler into the tunnel, and rest it on the anterior surface of the artery (Figure 12-10). *Once in position, the stapler is not moved. This is a key maneuver.*
- While the stapler is held steady, pull the lung parenchyma into the stapler. After adequate advancement has been made, fire the stapler. Normally, use a green load stapler to complete the fissure; however, if the fissure is well developed and there is not much lung parenchyma to be stapled, use a vascular load.
- Continue this process of opening the fissure by creating the tunnel until the fissure is completed. The pulmonary artery and the bronchus should be clearly visualized.
- With this view, the left lower lobe (LLL) bronchus is seen running underneath the artery. The lingular artery and the left upper lobe bronchus are seen to the left of the screen traveling to the upper lobe. The basilar trunk arteries and the LLL bronchus are seen going to the right of the screen to the lower lobe (Figure 12-11).

Step 7: Transecting the Pulmonary Artery

- **Exposure:** The exposure is not changed.
- The camera angle is not changed.
- With the Metzenbaum scissors through the lower anterior incision, dissect between the LLL bronchus and the lower lobe artery.
- When the artery has been almost completely mobilized, isolate the artery with the right-angle clamp brought through the utility incision.
- Usually, with one firing of the vascular stapler, all branches of the lower lobe artery can be transected. Occasionally, the superior segmental branch is addressed separately.
- If it is difficult to pass the stapler around the artery, lift the artery with a tie, or pass a red (rubber) Robinson-Nelaton (Rob-Nel) catheter to guide the stapler (Figure 12-12).
- The lower anterior incision provides the best angle for the stapler to transect the lower lobe pulmonary artery.

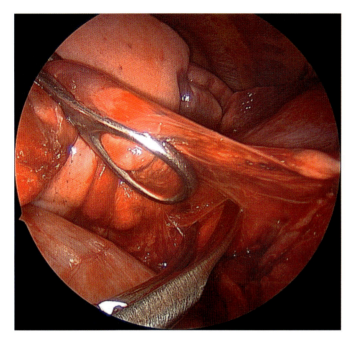

Figure 12-9. To complete the remainder of the fissure, a tunnel is created on the surface of the artery with blunt or sharp dissection. The anvil of the tissue stapler is placed in this tunnel (see Figure 12-10).

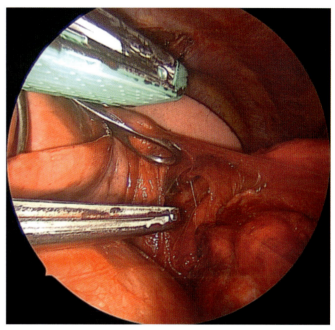

Figure 12-10. The anvil rests on the surface of the pulmonary artery and is kept stationary; this is critical. Lung parenchyma is then fed into the stapler. The stapler is fired, and this step is repeated as many times as necessary to complete the fissure.

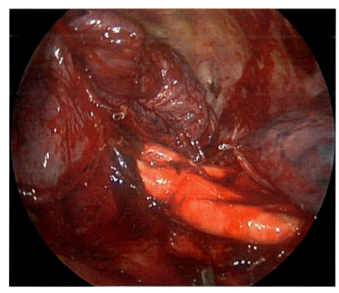

Figure 12-11. After the fissure is completely opened, branches of the pulmonary artery and the left lower lobe bronchus are clearly identified.

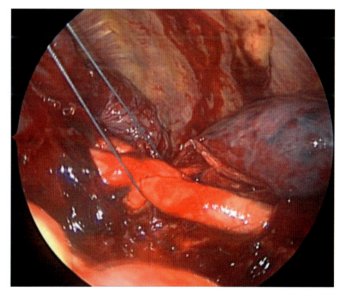

Figure 12-12. Occasionally, a tie around the lower lobe branches of the pulmonary artery facilitates passage of the vascular stapler.

Step 8: Transection of the Bronchus
- **Exposure:** Pull the LLL inferiorly and laterally.
- Aim the 30-degree lens superiorly and medially.
- At this point, the lower lobe bronchus is all that attaches the LLL to the patient (Figure 12-13).
- Transect the bronchus with a tissue stapler, which is brought through the lower anterior incision (Figure 12-14).
- The LLL is fully disconnected.

Step 9. Lobe Removal
- The lobe is removed, and the node dissection is completed.
- The technique for left-sided mediastinal lymph node dissection is reviewed in Chapter 22.

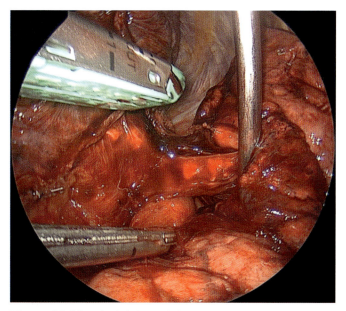

Figure 12-13. The left lower lobe bronchus is the only remaining structure.

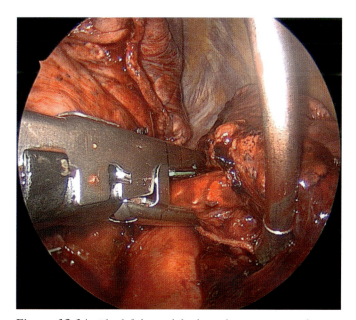

Figure 12-14. The left lower lobe bronchus is transected.

CHAPTER 13

SLEEVE LOBECTOMY: RIGHT UPPER LOBE — VIDEO 13

Robert J. McKenna, Jr.

Introduction

Surgeons with excellent video skills can perform a standard sleeve lobectomy as video-assisted thoracic surgery (VATS). The initial steps for a right upper lobe (RUL) sleeve lobectomy are the same as for a standard right upper lobectomy.

Approach to Video-Assisted Sleeve Lobectomy of the Right Upper Lobe

Order of Operative Steps

The order of the steps of the operation is as follows: level 10 nodes, RUL vein, anterior trunk of the artery, minor fissure, posterior ascending artery, and the fissure. The mainstem and the intermediate bronchi are then cut. The bronchial anastomosis is made through the utility incision with standard thoracotomy instruments. The standard incisions are used, with the utility incision placed directly up (lateral) from the superior pulmonary vein.

Key Points

- Use the standard approach for a right upper lobectomy initially.
- The right upper lobe bronchus is posterior to the right pulmonary artery and must be separated from the artery for transection.
- Mediastinoscopy with a complete subcarinal node dissection mobilizes the mainstem and intermediate bronchi from the lymph nodes and pericardium. Perform the mediastinoscopy during the same anesthesia as the sleeve lobectomy because a delay between the two procedures produces adhesions that make the dissection more difficult.
- At the junction of the cartilage and membranous portion of the intermediate bronchus, place a stay suture posteriorly to help appose the intermediate and mainstem bronchi.
- Place the posterior row of sutures first.

Video-Assisted Sleeve Lobectomy of the Right Upper Lobe (Video 13)

Step 1. Initial Procedures
- Address the level 10 nodes, right upper lobe vein, and fissure as described for a standard right upper lobectomy in Chapter 8.

Step 2. Transection of Bronchi
- **Exposure:** Retract the lung posteriorly and slightly inferiorly (Figure 13-1).
- Aim the thoracoscope anteriorly with the 30-degree lens pointed posteriorly.
- With a knife on a long handle through the utility incision, cut the mainstem and intermediate bronchi. Usually cut the bronchi from anterior to posterior so the cut is made away from the pulmonary artery (Figure 13-2).

Step 3. Posterior Bronchial Anastomosis
- **Exposure:** Retract the lung posteriorly and slightly inferiorly.
- Aim the thoracoscope anteriorly with the 30-degree lens pointed posteriorly.
- Retract the RUL posteriorly and apically with a ring forceps through incision 4.
- Place a stay suture posteriorly on the intermediate bronchus to help approximate the intermediate and mainstem bronchi (Figure 13-3).
- It is not necessary to take down the inferior pulmonary ligament for a routine RUL, but it does help take tension off the anastomosis for a sleeve resection.
- Place the interrupted sutures from posterior to anterior along the membranous portion on the bronchus with a standard needle holder through the utility incision (Figure 13-4).[1]
- Tie the knots inside or outside the lumen. Tie the knots as the sutures are placed because placing the sutures first and tying the knots later creates a very difficult task of keeping the sutures in order and preventing them from becoming crossed as later sutures are placed.

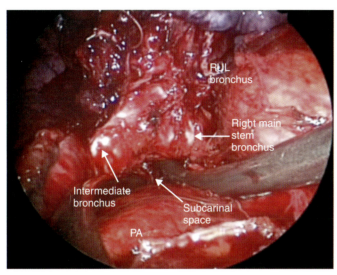

Figure 13-1. The suction catheter in the subcarinal space exposes the bronchus for transection. *PA,* Pulmonary artery; *RUL,* right upper lobe.

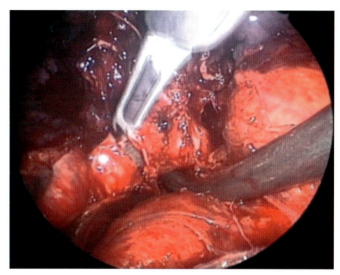

Figure 13-2. The intermediate bronchus is transected with a knife on a long handle.

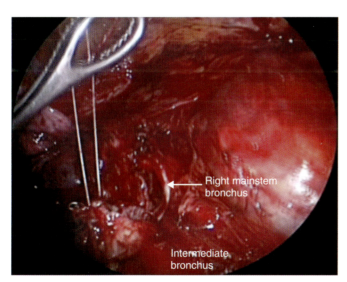

Figure 13-3. The stay suture is placed posteriorly in the intermediate bronchus.

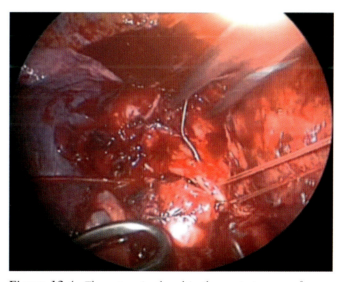

Figure 13-4. The suture is placed in the posterior row of sutures.

4. Completion of Bronchi Anastomosis

- **Exposure:** Retract the lung posteriorly and slightly inferiorly.
- Aim the thoracoscope anteriorly with the 30-degree lens pointed posteriorly.
- Place the sutures for the remainder of the anastomosis so the knots are tied outside the lumen (Figure 13-5).
- The anastomosis is close enough to a properly placed utility incision so the knots may be tied extracorporeally and then pushed with a finger through the utility incision to the anastomosis. Rarely, a knot pusher is needed.
- Fill the chest with water (not saline) because the red blood cells explode in water, allowing better visualization through the water to examine the anastomosis for possible bleeding or air leak.
- Perform fiberoptic bronchoscopy at the conclusion of the anastomosis to confirm that the anastomosis is not narrowed and to remove any blood clots in the bronchial tree.

Postoperative Care

- Provide standard postoperative care for patients after a lobectomy.
- Have a low threshold for a therapeutic bronchoscopy, because after the bronchus has been completely transected, the bronchial cilia do not work normally to help remove mucus.

Reference

1. Mahtabifard A, Fuller CB, McKenna RJ Jr: VATS sleeve lobectomy, *Ann Thorac Surg* 85:S729–S732, 2008.

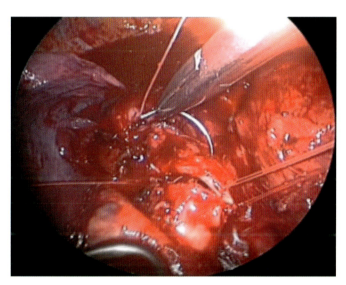

Figure 13-5. The anterior row of sutures is placed.

CHAPTER 14

SLEEVE LOBECTOMY: RIGHT MIDDLE LOBE SUPERIOR SEGMENT— VIDEO 14

Robert J. McKenna, Jr.

Introduction

Surgeons with excellent video skills can perform a standard sleeve lobectomy as video-assisted thoracic surgery (VATS). When a tumor involves the origin of the middle lobe bronchus and the intermediate bronchus or involves the origin of the superior segmental lobe bronchus and the intermediate bronchus, a sleeve lobectomy of the middle lobe and the superior segment of the lower lobe may be a good parenchyma-sparing operation that provides good margins around the tumor. A carcinoid tumor in this location may be a good indication for this procedure, which would avoid a pneumonectomy.

Approach to Video-Assisted Sleeve Lobectomy of the Right Middle Lobe Superior Segment

Order of Operative Steps

The order of the steps of the operation is as follows: right middle lobe (RML) vein, middle lobe artery, minor fissure, major fissure between the middle lobe and the lower lobe, superior segment separated from the basilar segments, superior segmental artery, the major fissure between the superior segment and the posterior segment of the right upper lobe, transecting the intermediate bronchus and the bronchus for the basilar segments, and anastomosis of the basilar segmental bronchus to the intermediate bronchus.

Key Points

- Use the standard approach for a RML initially, including the incisions shown in Figure 14-1.
- Place a stay suture posteriorly on the basilar segmental bronchus because it retracts into the lower lobe parenchyma and helps oppose the basilar segmental bronchi and the intermediate bronchus.
- Take down the inferior pulmonary ligament to minimize tension on the anastomosis.
- Place the posterior row of sutures first.

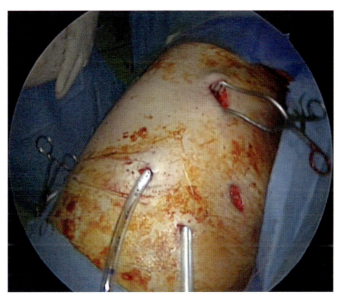

Figure 14-1. Incisions for a sleeve lobectomy of the right middle lobe superior segment.

Video-Assisted Sleeve Lobectomy of the Right Middle Lobe Superior Segment

Step 1. Right Middle Lobe Vein

- **Exposure:** Retract the lung directly posteriorly.
- The thoracoscope is aimed anteriorly with the 30-degree lens pointed posteriorly toward the hilum.
- Dissect between the inferior and superior pulmonary veins to define the inferior border of the RML vein and to determine whether there is drainage from the middle lobe to the inferior pulmonary vein (Figure 14-2).
- With DeBakey pickups and Metzenbaum scissors, define the superior aspect of the RML vein.
- Pass a right-angle clamp through the utility incision around the RML vein (Figure 14-3).
- With the vascular endoscopic stapler introduced from the utility incision or the auscultatory incision, transect the RML vein.

Step 2. Middle Lobe Artery

- **Exposure:** Retract the lung posteriorly.
- The thoracoscope is aimed anteriorly with the 30-degree lens pointed posteriorly.
- The RML artery parallels the bronchus and is located just superior and slightly medial to the bronchus (Figure 14-4).
- With Metzenbaum scissors, separate the artery from the bronchus.
- Pass a right-angle clamp around the artery and spread widely.
- Tie or double clip the artery (Figures 14-5 and 14-6).

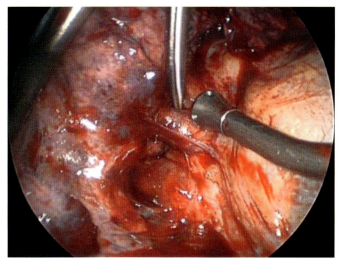

Figure 14-2. Exposure for the right middle lobe vein, superior pulmonary vein, and inferior pulmonary vein.

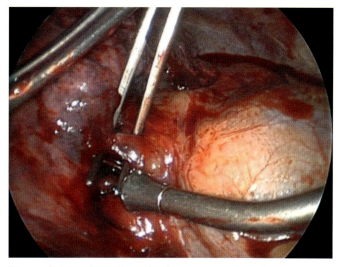

Figure 14-3. The right-angle clamp passes around the right middle lobe vein.

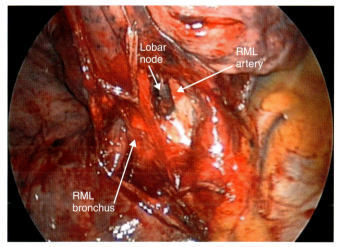

Figure 14-4. Relationship of the right middle lobe (RML) bronchus and artery.

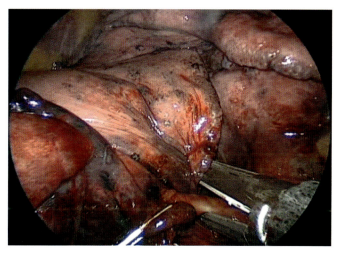

Figure 14-5. Clips on the right middle lobe artery.

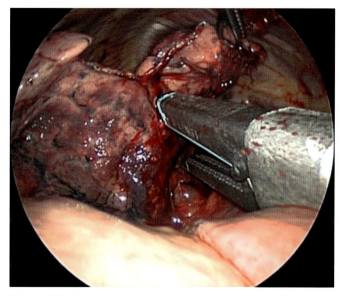

Figure 14-6. The anvil of the stapler is on the artery, and the stapler is held in that position.

Step 3. Minor Fissure

- **Exposure:** Retract the middle lobe posteriorly and slightly inferiorly.
- The thoracoscope is aimed anteriorly with the 30-degree lens pointed posteriorly.
- Identify the minor fissure.
- Pull the middle lobe and upper lobe inferiorly to line up the minor fissure with incision 1 or incision 3.
- If the fissure is thick, compress the lung parenchyma with a ring forceps.
- Pass the stapler (with a blue or green load cartridge) through either incision toward the lung. Carefully point the anvil of the stapler toward the space between the middle lobe and upper lobe veins. If the stapler is pointed more obliquely, it can tear into the lung parenchyma. Fire the stapler.
- For the second firing of the stapler, place the anvil on the pulmonary artery in the space between the confluence of the middle and upper lobe veins. With the ring forceps, pull the lung parenchyma into the stapler (Figure 14-7).

Step 4. Major Fissure between the Middle Lobe and the Lower Lobe

- **Exposure:** Retract the right lower lobe (RLL) posteriorly and slightly inferiorly, and retract the RML inferiorly and anteriorly to line up the major fissure with the stapler.
- The thoracoscope is aimed anteriorly with the 30-degree lens pointed posteriorly.
- For most patients who have a parenchymal bridge of tissue that extends for the entire length of the major fissure, pass the stapler through incision 1, and point it directly up the major fissure. The first firing of the stapler is safe because the device cannot reach the artery in the fissure (Figure 14-8).
- Lift the parenchyma in the fissure with a ring forceps. The artery and the bronchus run parallel to each other (Figure 14-9). Remove the lobar node between the RLL and RML bronchus to better define the artery. Spread the Metzenbaum scissors on the surface of the artery to create a tunnel.
- Place the anvil of the stapler on the artery in the tunnel. Pull lung parenchyma into the stapler to complete the major fissure between the RML and the RLL (Figure 14-10).
- If the connection between the RML and the RLL in the major fissure does not extend to the inferior aspect of the major fissure, completion of this part of the fissure begins with lifting the parenchyma of the fissure to find the artery.

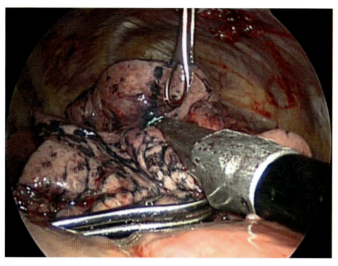

Figure 14-7. The ring forceps pulls the lung tissue into the jaws of the stapler, and the stapler remains stable. The relation of the anvil to the artery does not change.

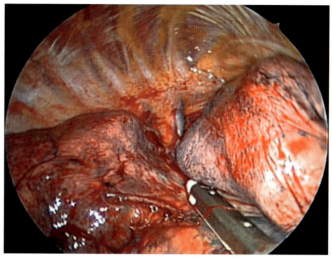

Figure 14-8. The stapler completes the fissure between the right middle lobe and the right lower lobe.

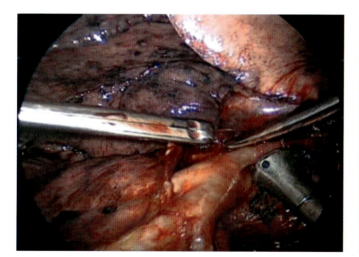

Figure 14-9. A ring forceps lifts the tissue in the major fissure to expose the right lower lobe bronchus and artery. The Metzenbaum scissors spreads tissue on the surface of the artery to create a tunnel for the stapler.

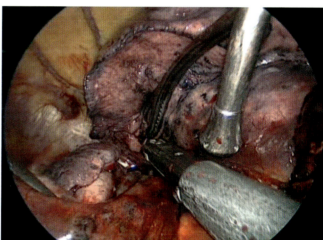

Figure 14-10. The stapler is used to complete the major fissure.

Step 5. Separating the Superior Segment from the Basilar Segments

* **Exposure:** Retract the RLL posteriorly and slightly inferiorly, and retract the RML inferiorly and slightly medially.
* The thoracoscope is aimed anteriorly with the 30-degree lens pointed posteriorly and apically.
* The dissection along the artery to complete the major fissure between the RML and the RLL exposes the RLL artery and the superior segmental artery. That landmark separates the superior segment from the basilar segments. There is often at least a small suggestion of a fissure at the inferolateral border of the superior segment.
* Direct the anvil of the stapler between the inferior border of the superior segmental artery and the RLL artery, and align the staple cartridge with the superior segmental fissure (Figure 14-11). Pull the lung parenchyma into the stapler. It usually needs to be fired three or four times to separate the superior segment (Figure 14-12).

Step 6. Superior Segmental Artery

* **Exposure:** Retract the RLL posteriorly, and retract the superior segment superiorly.
* The thoracoscope is aimed anteriorly with the 30-degree lens pointed posteriorly and apically.
* With the superior segment separated, the superior segmental artery is seen, and the superior segmental bronchus is posterior to the bronchus.
* Mobilize the superior segmental artery for clipping or stapling (Figures 14-13 and 14-14).

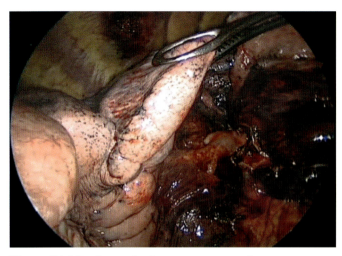

Figure 14-11. The stapler begins to separate the superior segment from the basilar segments.

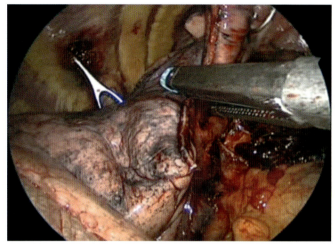

Figure 14-12. The anvil of the stapler is pointed between the right lower lobe artery and the artery for the superior segment.

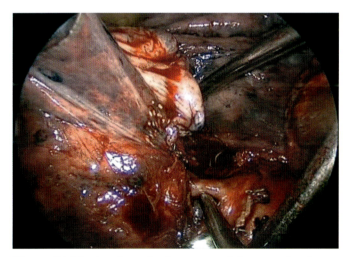

Figure 14-13. A right-angle clamp around the artery for the superior segment of the right lower lobe mobilizes it so that it can be clipped.

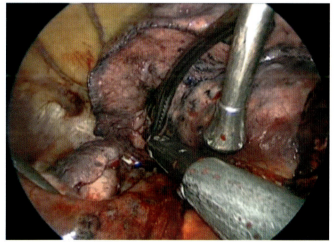

Figure 14-14. The right middle lobe and superior segments are retracted inferiorly. The Metzenbaum scissors is used to dissect on the surface of the artery to create a tunnel for the stapler to complete the fissure between the posterior segment of the right upper lobe and the superior segment of the right lower lobe.

Step 7. Completing the Major Fissure between the Superior Segment and the Posterior Segment of the Right Upper Lobe

- **Exposure:** Retract the lung posteriorly and slightly inferiorly.
- The thoracoscope is aimed anteriorly with the 30-degree lens pointed posteriorly.
- At this point in the operation, the superior segment and the middle lobe are attached, and they surround the artery. Transect the lung parenchyma as far from the tumor as possible.
- If the tumor is by the middle lobe bronchus and does not involve the major fissure, complete the entire major fissure by continuing to dissect along the surface of the artery to create a tunnel for the stapler.
- If the tumor is by the superior segmental bronchus and does come close to or involve the major fissure, transect the RML bronchus with a stapler.
- Complete the major fissure between the RLL superior segment and the right upper lobe (RUL) posterior segment (Figure 14-15). Complete the minor fissure to expose the artery in the fissure. With the Metzenbaum scissors, dissect transversely between the posterior ascending artery and the artery for the superior segment.
- Place the anvil of the stapler on the artery, and pull the parenchyma of the major fissure into the stapler.

Step 8. Transecting the Intermediate Bronchus and the Bronchus for the Basilar Segments

- **Exposure:** Retract the lung posteriorly and slightly inferiorly.
- The thoracoscope is aimed anteriorly with the 30-degree lens pointed posteriorly.
- The bronchus lies posterior and medial to the artery. With sharp and blunt dissection, separate the two structures (Figure 14-16).
- Retract the artery anteriorly to expose and transect the basilar segmental bronchus at the inferior margin of the superior segmental bronchus. With a scalpel, cut the mainstem and intermediate bronchi. It may be safer to cut the bronchi from anterior to posterior so that the cut is made away from the artery (Figure 14-17).
- Place a stay suture on the basilar segmental bronchus before it is completely transected, because it retracts into the lung tissue.

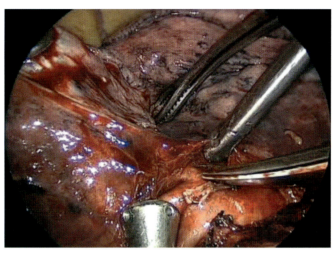

Figure 14-15. The stapler is completing the major fissure between the right upper lobe posterior segment and the right lower lobe superior segment.

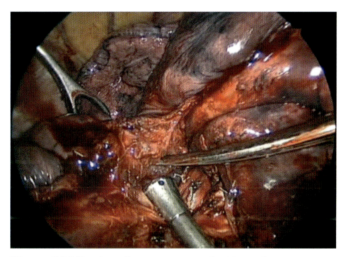

Figure 14-16. Blunt dissection using the Metzenbaum scissors separates the right lower lobe artery and bronchus.

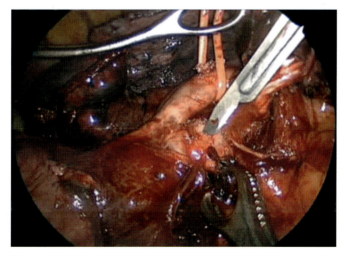

Figure 14-17. The scalpel is used to cut the basilar segmental bronchus.

Step 9. Posterior Bronchial Anastomosis

* **Exposure:** Retract the lung posteriorly and slightly inferiorly.
* The thoracoscope is aimed anteriorly with the 30-degree lens pointed posteriorly.
* With a ring forceps from incision 4, retract the RUL posteriorly and apically.
* Place a stay suture posteriorly on the intermediate bronchus to help approximate the intermediate and the mainstem bronchi (Figure 14-18).
* Take down the inferior pulmonary ligament to take tension off the anastomosis for a sleeve resection.
* Using a standard needle holder through the utility incision (4), place the interrupted sutures from posterior to anterior along the membranous portion on the bronchus (Figure 14-19).
* Tie the knots inside or outside the lumen. It is better to tie the knots as the sutures are placed, because placing the sutures first and tying the knots later requires keeping the sutures in order and preventing them from becoming crossed as the sutures are placed.

Step 10. Completion of the Bronchial Anastomosis

* **Exposure:** Retract the lung posteriorly and slightly inferiorly.
* The thoracoscope is aimed anteriorly with the 30-degree lens pointed posteriorly.
* Place the sutures for the remainder of the anastomosis, and tie the knots on the outside of the bronchial wall (Figure 14-20).
* Tie the knots extracorporeally, and push the knots with a finger through the utility incision. Rarely, a knot pusher is needed.
* Fill the chest with water (not saline), because the red blood cells explode in the water. That allows better visualization through the water to examine the anastomosis for possible bleeding or an air leak.
* Fiberoptic bronchoscopy at the conclusion of the anastomosis is important to confirm that the anastomosis is not narrowed and to remove any blood that went into the bronchial tree when the bronchus was open.

Step 11. Specimen Removal

* Remove the specimen as described in Chapter 5.

Postoperative Care

* Provide standard postoperative care for patients after a lobectomy.
* Maintain a low threshold for a therapeutic bronchoscopy, because after the bronchus has been completely transected, the bronchial cilia do not work normally to help remove mucus.

Reference

1. Mahtabifard A, Fuller CB, McKenna RJ Jr: VATS sleeve lobectomy, *Ann Thorac Surg* 85:S729–S732, 2008.

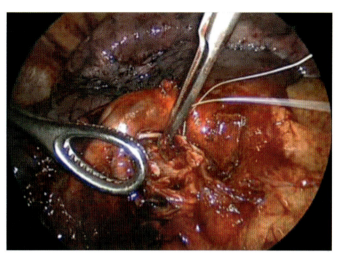

Figure 14-18. The stay suture approximates the basilar segmental bronchus and the intermediate bronchus.

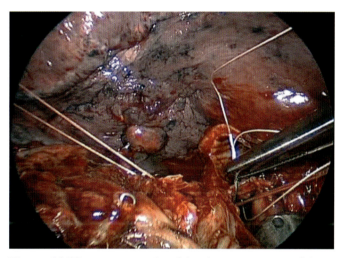

Figure 14-19. A suture is placed for the posterior row of the anastomosis.

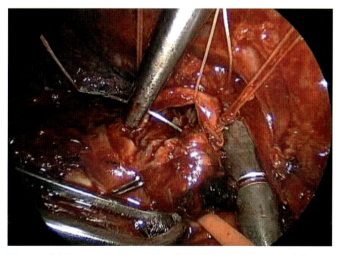

Figure 14-20. A suture is placed for the anterior row of the anastomosis.

CHAPTER 15

ROBOT–ASSISTED RIGHT UPPER LOBECTOMY

James T. Wu and Kemp H. Kernstine

Introduction

The da Vinci system (Intuitive Surgical, Sunnyvale, Calif) has three components: an operating console for the surgeon; a praying mantis–like chassis, from which spring the robotic video unit and the three robotic arms; and the electronic communication tower system between the console and the chassis (Figure 15-1).

Approach to Robot-Assisted Right Upper Lobectomy

Order of Operative Steps

The order of the steps of the operation is as follows: patient positioning, port placement, docking, right upper lobe (RUL) vein, RUL pulmonary artery, RUL bronchus, and minor fissure.

Key Points

- A thoracotomy tray should be in the operating room at all times.
- A ring clamp with a heavy sponge or Surgicel attached should be available for immediate use (Figure 15-2).
- Continuous intrathoracic carbon dioxide (CO_2) insufflation is used to enhance the robotically assisted surgery. Keep the intrathoracic CO_2 pressure less than 10–15 mm Hg to minimize a decrease in venous return and cardiac compliance.
- Avoid grasping the lung, hilar structures, or the airway with robotic instruments to minimize the risk of injury and bleeding. Non-robotic, less traumatic instruments are recommended to grasp the lung and will be discussed later in this chapter. The robotic instruments used are better suited for sweeping and very precise grasping.

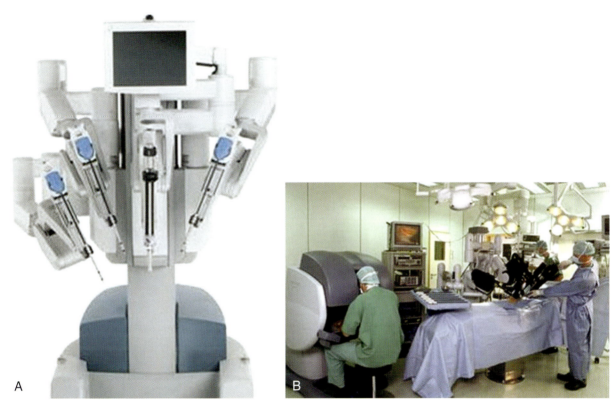

Figure 15-1. **A**, The Intuitive da Vinci System. **B**, is demonstrated in the typical operating room setup.

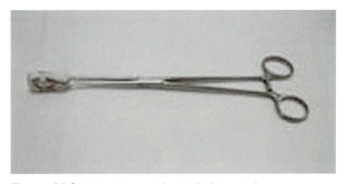

Figure 15-2. Ring clamp with attached Surgicel.

Robot-Assisted Right Upper Lobectomy

Step 1. Patient Positioning

- The patient is placed in the lateral decubitus and reversed Trendelenburg position (Figure 15-3). This allows the diaphragm and intra-abdominal contents to drop away from the operative field to increase exposure and allows any bleeding that occurs to pool away from the operative field.
- The patient's bed position is rotated 15 to 30 degrees posteriorly, and the head of the patient is directed toward the robotic chassis.

Step 2. Port Placement

- The four, 10- to 12-mm thoracoports (A, C, D, and F) are placed as shown in Figure 15-4.
- The target is the hilum, and the approximate location is drawn onto the patient's chest; this is a 4-cm-diameter circle whose center is approximately 3 cm anterior and 2 cm cephalad to the tip of the scapula.
- The camera port (A) is placed in the eighth or ninth intercostal space (ICS) adjacent to the anterior costal margin. After the port is slowly placed in position, the pleural space is visualized to ensure there has been no damage to intrathoracic structures.
- CO_2 is slowly infused to pressures of 10 to 15 mm Hg. If there is no evidence of pleural metastatic disease, the remaining thoracoports are placed.
- Place the thoracoports under direct intrapleural visualization to avoid injury to the neurovascular bundles and postoperative neuralgia.
- The most anterosuperior port site, usually in the anterior axillary to lateral clavicular line in the fourth ICS, serves as the utility port (F).
- The inferoanterior port, located in the anterior axillary line in the eighth to ninth ICS (B) and another port located in the posterior axillary line in the eighth to ninth ICS (E) are 8-mm ports used for the robotic arms. Both robotic ports are placed 10 to 12 cm on a lateral plane away from the camera port (A).
- The superoposterior site is marked at roughly the fourth ICS posteriorly about 8 to 10 cm from the posterior spinous processes so that it enters the chest at or just below the posterior aspect of the major fissure (D).
- The inferoposterior port site is located at the tenth ICS along the same longitudinal line as the superoposterior port site (C).
- Both posterior ports (D and C) are often placed just lateral to the longitudinal spinous muscle to allow passage of staplers and introduction of suctioning and retracting equipment.

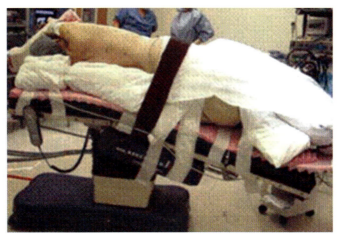

Figure 15-3. The patient is placed in the lateral decubitus position with a supporting axillary roll. In a patient with large hips, a slight reverse bend at the midportion of the table helps to move the hips out of the way.

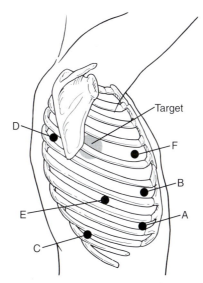

Figure 15-4. Port placement for the right upper lobectomy. Four, 10- to 12-mm thoracoports (A, C, D, F) are placed. The inferoanterior port (B) and another port (E) are used for the robotic arms. Both robotic ports are placed 10 to 12 cm from the camera port (A).

Step 3. Docking

- Roll the robot into position approximately 30 degrees from directly over the head and in line with the camera port and the target (Figure 15-5).
- After the chassis is locked into the correct distance from the operating table, compress the setup button to pull the robotic arms into position.
- Latch the video arm and robotic arms onto their respective ports.
- Insert the videoscope into the thoracic cavity under direct vision.
- Instrument choice depends on the surgeon. We prefer using the ProGrasp instrument in the left arm and the Harmonic scalpel or Hook electrocautery in the right arm.
- A Landreneau ring grasper is placed into the superoposterior port (see Figure 15-4, port D) to grasp the upper lobe just superior to the hilar location. The grasper is allowed to rest under gravity, providing sufficient lateral traction.

Step 4. Right Upper Lobe Vein

- **Exposure:** Direct the camera toward the upper anterior hilum.
- The videoscope is either the 0- or 30-degree scope in the down position. When interchanging scopes, 0- and 30-degree, make sure to adjust the view parameters at the console.
- The Harmonic scalpel divides the mediastinal tissue and pleura adjacent to the phrenic nerve up to the level of the upper hilum and azygous vein.
- Use the ProGrasp forceps to sweep the tissue cleanly away from the proximal pulmonary vein.
- Identify the bifurcation between the right middle and right upper lobe veins. The hilar lymphatic tissue between the middle and upper lobe veins is bluntly cleaned and lifted away from the intermedius and middle lobe pulmonary arteries.
- Bluntly sweep the hilar tissue toward the resection specimen, clearing the pulmonary artery and under aspect of the RUL vein.
- Blunt and Harmonic scalpel dissection clears away the tissue from the azygous vein and continues the en bloc dissection to the main pulmonary artery.
- Pass an 8-cm, 0 silk tie around the vein to retract it away from the pulmonary artery beneath it.
- Passed from the inferoposterior port site, an endostapler is used to transect the RUL vein (Figure 15-6).

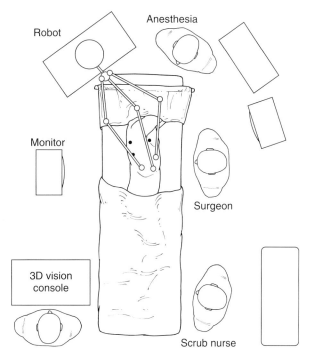

Figure 15-5. Positioning of the robot.

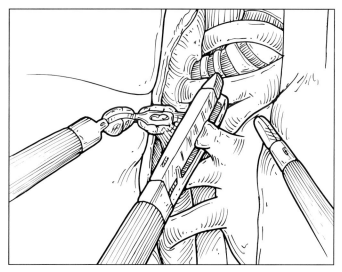

Figure 15-6. Division of the right upper lobe vein. The superior pulmonary vein of the right upper lobe is identified, and the adjacent nodal tissue is taken en bloc with it. Effort should be made to separate it from and preserve the middle lobe vein.

Step 5. Right Upper Lobe Pulmonary Artery

◆ **Exposure:** If necessary, regrasp the hilar tissue using the Landreneau clamp to provide better exposure of the main pulmonary artery and its branches.

◆ Use the ProGrasp forceps to sweep the hilar tissue off the cephalad aspect of the pulmonary artery to its junction so the middle lobe artery and the recurrent branch are cleanly exposed.

◆ Each branch can be identified at its origin and ligated with the vascular endostapler, exposing the nodes just anterior to the mainstem bronchus (Figure 15-7).

Step 6. Right Upper Lobe Bronchus

◆ **Exposure:** Prior to taking the bronchus and especially in cases when we do not have adequate 3-dimensional visualization of the bronchus, we like to visualize the posterior aspect of the hilum and sometimes perform some of the peribronchial dissection and exposure, especially when the tumors are close to the hilum or when there is an extensive amount of inflammation or fibrosis. To do so, release the Landreneau retractor to allow the right upper lobe to rotate anteriorly to expose the posterior hilum and airway.

◆ Divide the pleura over the posterior hilum, and sweep it toward the specimen.

◆ Identify the posterior aspect of the major fissure, and if not already separated, divide the posterior aspect of the major fissure by using the endostapler through the upper posterior port.

◆ Clear the bifurcation of the bronchus intermedius and the RUL bronchus with the ProGrasp forceps and the Harmonic scalpel. In this location, the subcarinal lymph nodes may be identified and resected. Dissected specimens are placed in an Endobag and brought out through one of the thoracoports.

◆ After the subcarinal nodes are removed, the attention is turned back to the anterior aspect of the main bronchus. The lung is again retracted posteriorly, and the Landreneau ring clamp from the posterosuperior port grasps the intended specimen.

◆ Now with the peribronchial hilar tissue sufficiently thinned, carefully pass the ProGrasp forceps behind the right upper lobe airway, and retract the bronchus with a silk tie to facilitate stapling (Figure 15 8).

◆ Through the posteroinferior thoracoport, pass around and close an endostapler passes, but do not fire it on the bronchus.

◆ To make certain that the correct airway has been identified, we perform two maneuvers. First, the anesthesiologist bronchoscopically examines the airway, and the surgeon visually confirms the location of the bronchoscope by the transilluminated light through the airway. Second, while the CO_2 insufflation is turned off, the remaining lung is inflated, confirming that it can inflate and deflate.

◆ After the bronchial transection, the hilum and mediastinum is flooded with irrigation fluid and the remaining lung inflated to 25 cm with H_2O to make certain there is no leak at the bronchial stump. If there is a leak, attempt to identify it and reinforce the bronchus with 2-3 carefully placed simple sutures of 4-0 prolene on an S-H needle cut to 8 cm length. Avoid strangulation of the tissue.

Step 7. Minor Fissure

◆ **Exposure:** The lung is retracted directly posteriorly and superiorly.

◆ An endoscopic stapler introduced through the anterosuperior port site completes the fissure. Identification of the middle lobe vein assists in identifying the anterior aspect of the minor fissure (Figure 15-9).

◆ After the fissure has been completed, the resected lobe is placed into the lower thorax, where it is out of the way for the next steps.

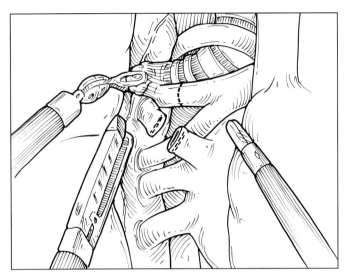

Figure 15-7. Division of the right upper lobe pulmonary artery. The hilar tissue is resected away from the right upper lobe pulmonary artery to expose it for transection.

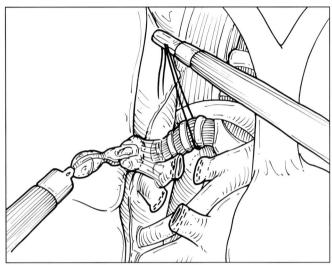

Figure 15-8. Division of the right upper lobe bronchus. After the division of the recurrent branch of the pulmonary artery to the right upper lobe and clearing of the hilar tissue between the right upper lobe and the bronchus intermedius, the right upper lobe bronchus is divided with an endostapler.

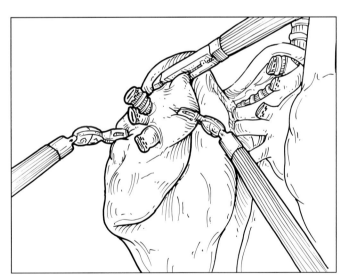

Figure 15-9. Division of the minor fissure of the right upper lobe. The endostapler is introduced through the anterosuperior thoracoport to divide the minor fissure, completing the right upper lobectomy.

Step 8. Lobe Removal

- **Exposure:** Adjust the camera as needed for optimal visualization.
- To prevent postoperative torsion of the right middle lobe in patients who have a near-complete fissure between the right middle and right lower lobes, a knifeless stapler attaches the most anteroinferior aspect of the right middle lobe to the most inferoanterior aspect of the right lower lobe.
- Insert a medium-sized Anchor bag into the apex of the chest through the anterosuperior thoracoport site (see Figure 15-4, port F). Prior to placing the Anchor bag, an intercostal incision with the robotic Hook Cautery is made about 6-7 cm in length along the intercostal where the most anterior superior port is located, the incision through which the specimen is to be removed. Avoid cauterizing the intercostal nerve and the rib periosteum.
- Place the lobe into the bag, and remove it.
- Turn off the CO_2, and vent the pleural space by opening up the air vents of each of the four ports.
- Remove the robotic instrument and arms.

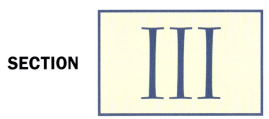

Segmentectomies

CHAPTER 16

LEFT UPPER LOBE APICAL TRISEGMENTECTOMY— VIDEO 16-1

Scott J. Swanson

Introduction

Segmentectomy is an option for a small, anatomically well-situated lung cancer. Creating the segmental fissure and dissecting out the segmental vessels can be done using a thoracoscopic technique. A left upper lobe apical trisegmentectomy (i.e., lingula-sparing left upper lobectomy) is similar to right upper lobectomy with preservation of the right middle lobe.

Approach to Video-Assisted Left Upper Lobe Apical Trisegmentectomy

Order of Operative Steps

The order of the steps of the operation is as follows: anterior, superior, and posterior pleurae over the hilum; upper division vein; anterior trunk; posterior artery; bronchus; and the fissure (Video 16-1).

Key Points

- The vessels help to determine the separation between the upper division and the lingula.
- Alternatively, the bronchus for the upper division can be divided and the lingula ventilated to determine where to place the staples to separate the upper division.

Video-Assisted Left Upper Lobe Apical Trisegmentectomy

Step 1. Port Placement (Figure 16-1)

- Place the camera port in the seventh intercostal space in the anterior axillary line; it can be modified depending on heart size.
- Place the access port in the fourth intercostal space in the mid-axillary line.
- Place the posterior port in the sixth intercostal space, just inferior to the tip of the scapula.

Step 2. Dissect Anterior Hilum and Aortopulmonary Window (Figure 16-2)

- **Exposure:** Retract the lung posteriorly through the posterior port.
- Place the thoracoscope in the camera port with the side arm to the left to look at anterior hilar structures.
- Dissect through the access port.
- Open the mediastinal pleura over the anterior hilum with an endokittner and the suction irrigator. This defines the venous drainage from the upper division of the left upper lobe (LUL). Dissect superiorly to the level of the aortopulmonary window.
- Removal of the level 5 nodes facilitates exposure of the vessels and prepares the superior and posterior aspect of the anterior trunk for subsequent transection.

Step 3. Open Posterior Mediastinal Pleura (Figure 16-3)

- **Exposure:** Retract the lung anteriorly through the access incision.
- Place the thoracoscope in the camera port with the side arm to the right.
- Open the posterior mediastinal pleura using blunt dissection with endokittners through the posterior port. Continue opening the pleural superiorly until the dissection connects with the posterior pleural opening with the anterior pleural dissection from steps 1 and 2.

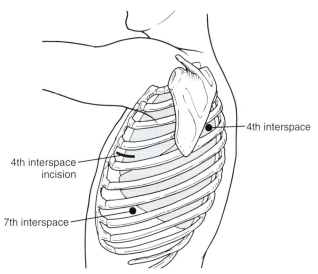

4th interspace

4th interspace
incision

7th interspace

Figure 16-1. The three ports for the left upper lobe apical trisegmentectomy are shown. The camera is placed in the seventh intercostal space in the anterior axillary line. The access port is in the fourth intercostal space in the mid-axillary line, and the posterior port is placed in the sixth intercostal space just inferior to the tip of the scapula.

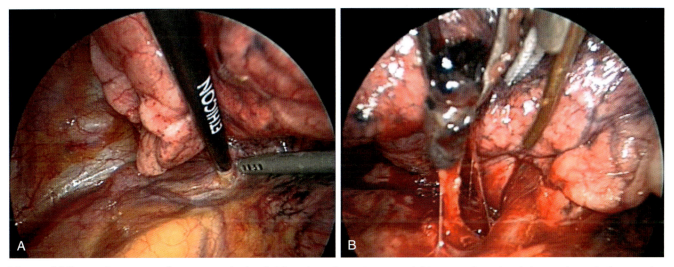

Figure 16-2. A, The surgeon dissects out the level 5 lymph nodes using an endokittner and suction irrigator through the anterior access port. The assistant gently retracts the lung posteriorly through the posterior port. **B,** The surgeon uses the harmonic scalpel to divide the small nodal vessels to the level 5 lymph nodes to ensure hemostasis through the anterior access port.

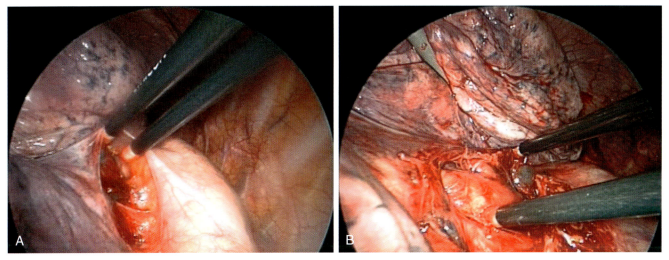

Figure 16-3. A, The lung is retracted anteriorly using a ring forceps through the anterior access port while the surgeon uses two endokittners through the posterior port to open the posterior mediastinal pleura, which exposes the level 6 lymph nodes, the vagus nerve, and the pulmonary artery where it enters the posterior fissure. **B,** The surgical assistant retracts the lung anteriorly through the anterior access port and uses the suction irrigator to further retract the lung. Suction as needed while the surgeon bluntly dissects out the pulmonary artery in the fissure using two endokittners through the posterior port.

Step 4. Tumor Palpation (Figure 16-4)

◆ **Exposure:** Move the lung toward the access port with a ringed forceps placed through the posterior port.
◆ Place the thoracoscope in the camera port with the side arm straight up.
◆ Carefully palpate and examine the tumor to be certain a sublobar resection constitutes optimal cancer treatment. This is done by corroborating the tumor size (T1, ideally less than 2 cm) and confirming that tumor is far enough away from the lingula so that the margins will be adequate if a trisegmentectomy is performed.
◆ When observing the LUL from an anterior position, the lingular vein helps to determine the superior aspect of the lingula. When retracting the LUL posteriorly, the upper division is just above the lingular vein. There is often a minimal fissure between the lingula and the upper division.

Step 5. Upper Pulmonary Vein (Figure 16-5)

◆ **Exposure:** Retract the lung posteriorly with the ring forceps through the posterior port.
◆ Place the thoracoscope in the camera port with the side arm to the left.
◆ Mobilize the upper division pulmonary vein with the endokittner and scissors or right-angle clamp. Carefully identify and preserve the lingular vein or veins. In some instances, it is necessary to divide a middle central vein, although it drains the upper division and lingula.

Step 6. Proximal Artery Dissection (Figure 16-6)

◆ **Exposure:** Retract the lung posteriorly and slightly inferiorly with ringed forceps through the posterior port.
◆ Place the thoracoscope through the camera port with the side arm to the left.
◆ Identify and dissect free the proximal artery with the endokittner and scissors placed through the camera port. Identify and mobilize the first and second branches. After the vein is divided, this dissection becomes easier.

Step 7. Dissection of the Pulmonary Artery in the Fissure (Figure 16-7)

◆ **Exposure:** Gently retract the lung superiorly and slightly anteriorly with the ringed forceps through the posterior port.
◆ Place the thoracoscope in the camera port with the side arm to the left.
◆ Identify the pulmonary artery in the fissure. Usually, this is easiest where the artery turns inferiorly to form the basilar trunk near the distal end of the fissure. Often, there is a lymph node sitting superficially over the artery at this point.
◆ Use two endokittners through the access incision to bluntly open the pleura over the artery in this location to establish the plane over the artery. When the proper plane is obtained, the white and glistening artery can be seen. Create a tunnel along the artery, extending it posteriorly toward the proximal pulmonary artery where it enters the fissure. The pulmonary artery was previously identified in this posterior location during steps 1 through 3. Divide the fissure with the endostapler to expose the upper lobe pulmonary artery branches.

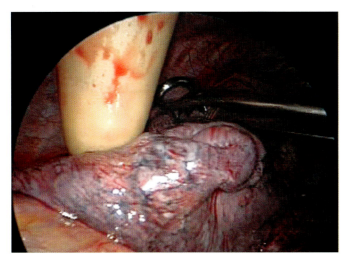

Figure 16-4. Through the anterior access port, the surgeon palpates the tumor to confirm its presence and determine that it is positioned centrally within the upper division.

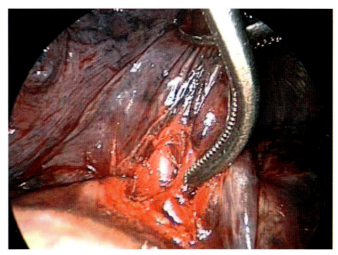

Figure 16-5. A right-angle clamp is passed around the upper division vein after it has been bluntly dissected free through the anterior access port. The assistant retracts the lung posteriorly through the posterior port.

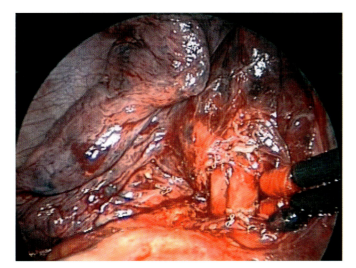

Figure 16-6. After division of the upper division vein, the surgeon dissects the first two branches of the left upper lobe artery through the camera port, with the camera shifted to the anterior access port before placing the vascular stapler.

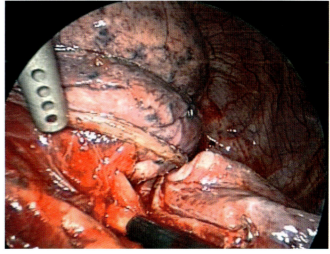

Figure 16-7. The surgeon dissects free the posterior segmental artery through the posterior port while the assistant retracts the lung anteriorly through the anterior access port with a ring forceps and suction irrigator.

Step 8. Upper Division Pulmonary Vein Division (Figure 16-8)

+ **Exposure:** Retract the lung posteriorly with ringed forceps through the posterior port.
+ Place the thoracoscope through the camera incision with the side arm to the left.
+ Before placing the stapler, use an endokittner through the posterior port to confirm that the stapler will pass at an appropriate angle and without undue tension.
+ Divide the upper division pulmonary vein using an endovascular stapler (white load cartridge, 30 to 45 mm) placed through the posterior port while retracting the lung with a ring forceps placed through the anterior port.

Step 9. Pulmonary Artery Division (Figure 16-9)

+ **Exposure:** Retract the lung posteriorly and inferiorly through the posterior port using a ringed forceps.
+ Place the thoracoscope through the access incision with the side arm straight up.
+ Divide the first and second branches of the pulmonary artery with the endovascular stapler placed through the camera port. Again test the angle of the proposed stapler placement using an endokittner.

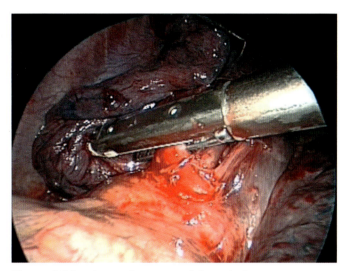

Figure 16-8. The stapler is passed through the posterior port around the upper division vein before dividing it.

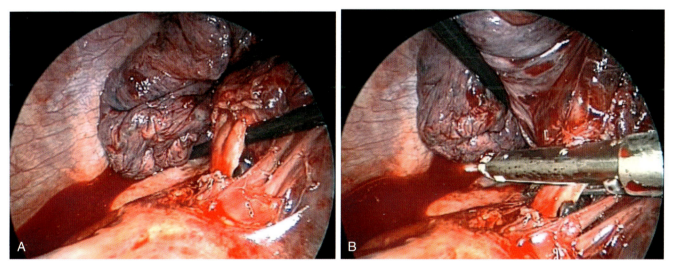

Figure 16-9. A, The endokittner passed through the camera port is placed around the first two branches of the left pulmonary artery to show that the vessel is free and that the angle of approach is appropriate for the straight vascular stapler. The camera is introduced through the anterior access port. **B,** Through the camera port, the vascular stapler is passed around the first two branches of the left pulmonary artery, with camera placed through the anterior access port. Alongside the camera, an endokittner is placed to retract the lung apically to allow excellent visualization of the stapler.

Step 10. Posterior Artery Division (Figure 16-10)

+ **Exposure:** Retract the lung anteriorly and apically with a ringed forceps through the access incision.
+ Place the thoracoscope through the camera incision with the side arm to the right.
+ Divide the posterior segmental artery with an endovascular stapler introduced through the posterior port. Because the first two pulmonary arterial branches have already been divided, the stapler should not be in danger of inadvertently injuring the branches.
+ The vascular stapler goes through the posterior incision.

Step 11. Bronchus Division (Figure 16-11)

+ **Exposure:** Retract the lung toward the anterior chest wall with a ringed forceps through the access incision to gain as much length on the bronchus as possible, and put it under some mild tension in the vertical plane.
+ Place the thoracoscope through the camera incision with the side arm to the right.
+ Dissect the posterior aspect of the bronchus.
+ Identify the upper division bronchus in the fissure, and sweep all peribronchial tissue up onto the bronchus with endokittners. This helps to identify the carina between the upper division bronchus and the lingular bronchus.
+ Dissect the anterior aspect of the bronchus. Retract the lung posteriorly with a ring forceps through the posterior port to bluntly dissect the same area from the anterior perspective using endokittners introduced through the access port. This helps to ensure that there is no tissue to impede the stapler.
+ Use an endobronchial stapler (blue or green load cartridge, 30 to 45 mm) placed through the posterior port to divide the upper division bronchus. Staple height is chosen based on the size of the segmental bronchus. If small, use a blue load; if bigger, use a green load. The same type of decision making is used for the length of the staples.

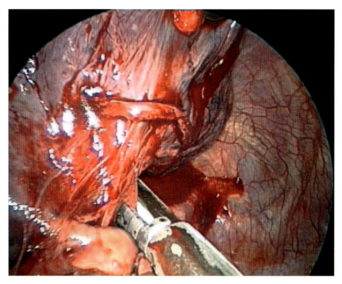

Figure 16-10. The vascular stapler is placed around the posterior segmental pulmonary artery through the posterior port. The lung is retracted with ringed forceps toward the anterior chest wall placed through the anterior access port along with an endokittner.

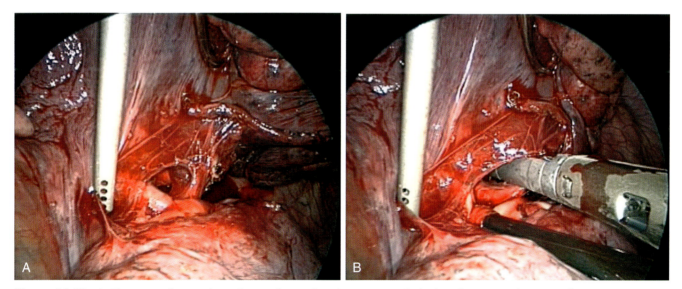

Figure 16-11. A, The upper division bronchus is observed in the center, with the lingular artery adjacent to the suction irrigator coursing anteriorly (toward the left side). **B,** The endostapler (blue load cartridge) is passed around the upper division bronchus through the posterior port alongside an endokittner. The lung is retracted with a ringed forceps through the anterior access port. A suction irrigator is passed through the same port for additional retraction and suction, as necessary.

Step 12. Complete the Fissure Between the Upper Division and the Lingula (Figure 16-12)

- **Exposure:** Retract the lung toward the anterior chest wall and slightly posteriorly with a ringed forceps through the posterior port.
- Place the thoracoscope through the camera incision with the side arm to the left.
- Divide the lung anteriorly between the stump of the upper division vein and lingular vein by placing the stapler (45- to 60-mm, gold or blue cartridge) through the access port while retracting the lung toward the anterior chest wall and slight posteriorly with a ring forceps placed through the posterior port. Occasionally, ring forceps are placed next to the stapler through the access port to aid in straightening the lung for stapled division.
- Divide the lung posteriorly between the divided posterior segmental artery and the intact lingular artery by placing the stapler (45- to 60-mm, gold or blue cartridge) through the posterior port while retracting the lung with a ring forceps placed through the access port. Place the camera in the camera port with the side arm to the right.
- Finish the fissure from anterior to posterior with a stapler (45- to 60-mm, gold or blue cartridge) through the posterior port. Retract the lung anteriorly toward the anterior chest wall and slightly posteriorly with a ring forceps placed through the access port. Be careful to keep the divided upper division bronchus up with the specimen and to avoid encroaching on the lingular bronchus. Before firing the stapler, the anesthesiologist should inflate the left lung to be sure the lingula inflates adequately. Place the camera through the camera port with the side arm to the left.

Step 13. Lapsac Retrieval (Figure 16-13)

- Specimen retrieval is described in Chapter 1.

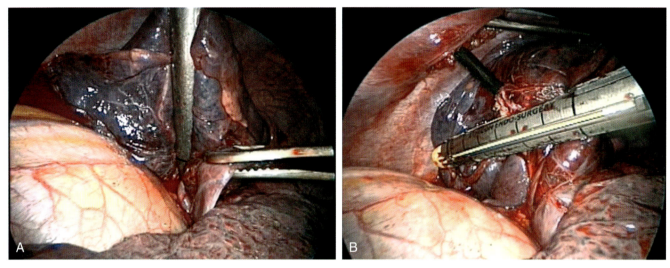

Figure 16-12. **A,** The anterior fissure between the upper division and the lingula is created with a stapler placed through the anterior access port. The lung is retracted with a ringed forceps through the posterior port. The surgeon must be careful to align the staple line parallel and just cephalad to the lingular vein. **B,** After beginning the fissure posteriorly, completion of the fissure is performed with the endostapler passed through the posterior port. The surgeon must be careful to avoid kinking or injuring the long, narrow lingular bronchus.

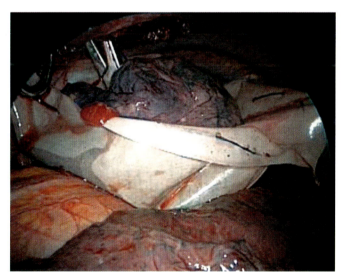

Figure 16-13. The specimen is placed in the Lapsac bag, which was brought in through the anterior access port after enlarging this incision to 5 cm.

Step 14. Inferior Pulmonary Ligament Takedown (Figure 16-14)
- **Exposure:** Retract the lung superiorly with a ring forceps placed through the posterior port.
- Place the thoracoscope through the camera incision with the side arm to the left.
- Take down the inferior pulmonary ligament with electrocautery through the access port while retracting the lung posteriorly and superiorly with a ring forceps through the posterior port.

Step 15. Subcarinal Node Dissection (Figure 16-15)
- Subcarinal node dissection is described in Chapter 22.

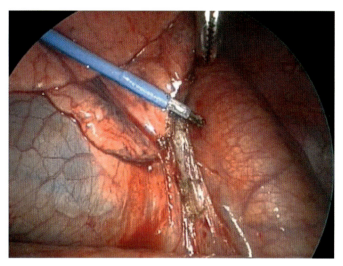

Figure 16-14. The inferior ligament is taken down with a long-handled electrocautery device introduced through the anterior access port. The lung is retracted cephalad through the posterior port with a ringed forceps.

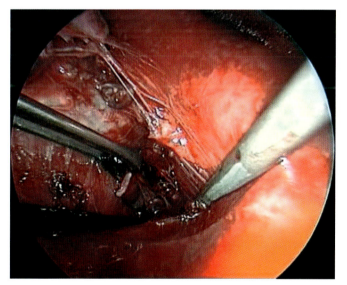

Figure 16-15. The subcarinal nodes are dissected free through the anterior access port with a long Allis clamp and endokittner. The esophagus and aorta are gently retracted posteriorly with the suction irrigator to aid in opening up this space. The left bronchus can be seen just posterior to the Allis clamp.

Step 16. Lung Inflation, Air Leak Check, and Placement of a Chest Tube (Figure 16-16)

- **Exposure:** Inflate the lung to see it expand, and test for an air leak.
- Place the thoracoscope through the camera incision with the side arm to the left or right side, depending on the best view.
- Reinflate the left lung to be sure that the lingula expands well and is positioned normally. Test the bronchial stump by instilling irrigation fluid with the suction irrigator and using a dental pledget to hold the lung down so the bronchial stump can be visualized. Place a single 24-French chest tube through the camera port posteriorly to the apex, and close remaining incisions.

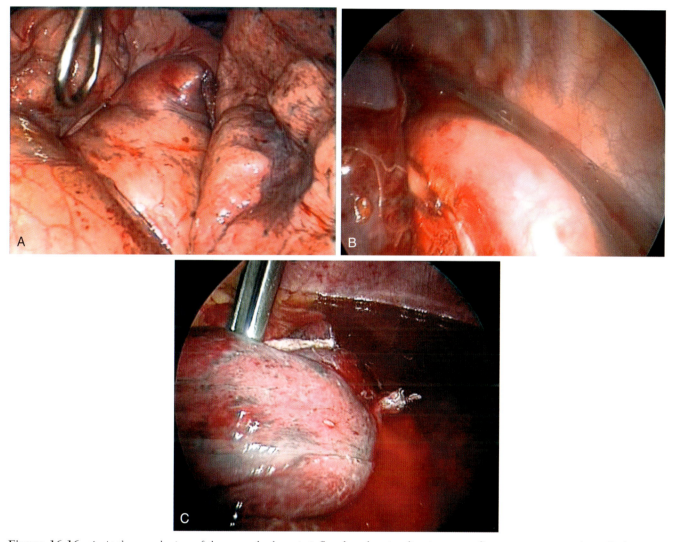

Figure 16-16. **A,** At the conclusion of the case, the lung is inflated under visualization to confirm a pneumostatic bronchial stump (irrigating fluid is introduced to submerge the bronchial stump) and ensure that the lingula expands well and is oriented properly. **B,** A 24-French chest tube is passed through the camera port posteriorly and toward the apex. Typically, an extra hole is created with a rongeur in the chest tube along the white radiopaque line at about 8 cm. **C,** The bronchial stump is submerged under saline introduced with the suction irrigator while the lung is inflated to test the stump.

CHAPTER 17

LINGULECTOMY—VIDEO 17

Robert J. McKenna, Jr.

Introduction

The anatomy of the lingua is consistent, and this operation is usually straightforward.

Approach to Video-Assisted Lingulectomy

Order of Operative Steps

The order of the steps for a lingulectomy is as follows: level 5 and 6 nodes, lingular vein, fissure, lingular artery, bronchus, and fissure.

Key Points

- A minimal fissure often can be identified between the lingula and upper division.
- Work from anterior to posterior.
- Rarely, the lingular veins can drain to both the superior pulmonary vein and the inferior pulmonary vein.

Video-Assisted Lingulectomy (Video 17)

Step 1. Incisions

- The standard incisions shown in Chapter 1 are used (see Figure 1-2).

Step 2. Resection of Level 5 and 6 Nodes

- The nodes are resected as for a left upper lobectomy (see Figure 11-1 in Chapter 11). This helps to define the anatomy of the superior pulmonary vein and branches.
- Rarely, the lingula may drain to the superior and inferior pulmonary veins.

Step 3. Lingular Vein

- **Exposure:** Retract the lung posteriorly through the posterior incision.
- Aim the thoracoscope slightly anteromedially, and point the lens slightly posteriorly.
- Look at the fissure and the superior pulmonary vein to identify the vein that drains the lingula.
- Through incision 3, dissect the vein from the lingula with DeBakey pickups and Metzenbaum scissors (Figure 17-1). Through the anterior incision, pass the right-angle clamp behind the vein, and spread it widely (Figure 17-2).
- Place clips through the anterior incision onto the lingular vein. Alternatively, staple the vein, but clips usually suffice because it is small (Figure 17-3).

Step 4. Complete the Fissure

- **Exposure:** Return the lung to its normal anatomic position. Through the posterior incision, retract the lower lobe posteriorly and inferiorly. Through the utility incision, retract the upper lobe anteriorly and superiorly.
- Aim the thoracoscope anteriorly, and point the 30-degree lens slightly inferiorly.
- If the fissure is incomplete, as is often the case, complete it with the stapler through incision 1. The stapler is well away from pulmonary artery (PA) in patients with an incomplete fissure.
- To complete more of the fissure, create a tunnel on the surface of the PA.
- Lift the lung parenchyma of the incomplete fissure away from the surface of the artery with a ring forceps (Figure 17-4).
- Identify the left upper lobe and the left lower lobe bronchi. Remove lymph nodes between the bronchi to expose the PA, which runs parallel to and on the surface of the left lower lobe bronchus.

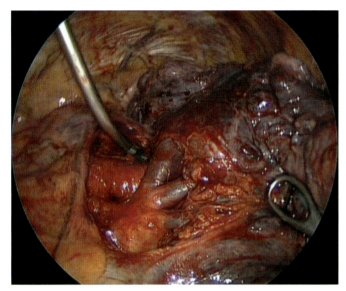

Figure 17-1. Superior vein, upper division vein, and lingular vein.

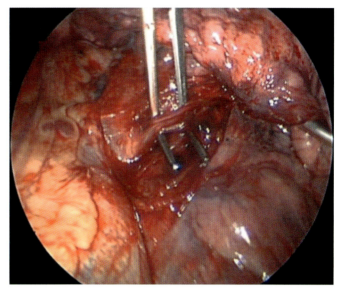

Figure 17-2. The right-angle clamp passes around the lingular vein.

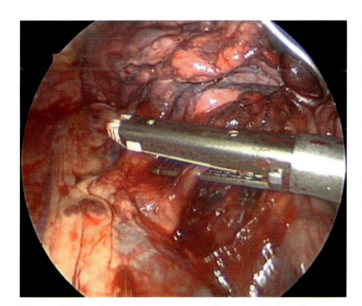

Figure 17-3. The stapler is positioned across the lingular vein.

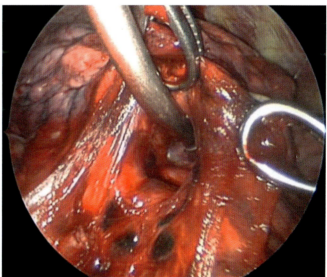

Figure 17-4. Exposure of the left upper lobe bronchus, left lower lobe bronchus, and the pulmonary artery that runs parallel to the lower lobe bronchus.

- With Metzenbaum scissors through incision 1, dissect on the surface of the PA to create a tunnel. Dissect on the lateral surface of the PA. As the dissection progresses, identify the lingular and posterior ascending arteries on the superior aspect of the PA. On the inferior side of the PA is the artery to the superior segment of the left lower lobe.
- Continue the dissection to just above the lingular artery. Complete the fissure with the stapler; the anvil of the stapler is placed into the tunnel and rests on the surface of the artery. Once in position, the stapler is not moved. This is a key maneuver (Figure 17-5).
- While the stapler is held in position, pull the lung parenchyma into the stapler with the ring forceps on the upper and lower lobes. Usually, a 4.8-mm stapler completes the fissure to just beyond the lingular artery. Use an avascular stapler for a thin fissure.
- This process of opening the fissure by creating the tunnel is repeated until the fissure is completed beyond the lingular artery.
- The left upper lobe bronchus, the main PA, and the lingular artery are readily identified.

Step 5. Lingular Artery
- **Exposure:** Retract the upper lobe superiorly and apically with a ring forceps through the anterior incision.
- Aim the thoracoscope anteriorly and slightly medially, and point the lens toward the mediastinum and slightly posteriorly.
- Bring the Metzenbaum scissors through incision 1 or 3 to dissect the lingular artery.
- With a right-angle clamp, completely mobilize the artery (Figure 17-6).
- Transect the artery with a vascular stapler through the inferior incision (Figure 17-7).

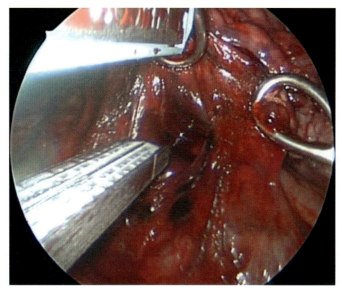

Figure 17-5. Placement of the anvil of the stapler to complete the fissure.

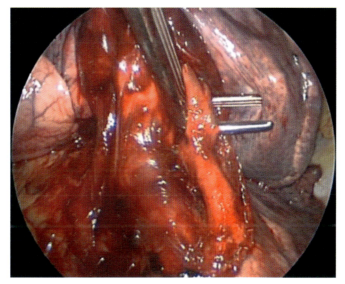

Figure 17-6. A right-angle clamp is used to mobilize the lingular artery.

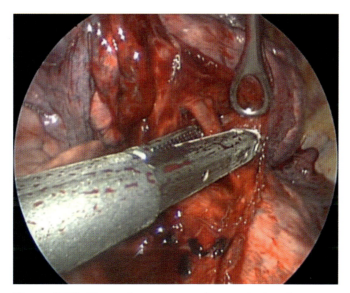

Figure 17-7. The stapler is positioned across the lingular artery.

Step 6. Lingular Bronchus

◆ **Exposure:** Retract the upper lobe superiorly and apically through the utility incision.
◆ Aim the thoracoscope anteriorly and slightly medially, and point the lens toward the mediastinum and slightly posteriorly.
◆ With the Metzenbaum scissors through incision 1 or 3, dissect the bronchus. With a right-angle clamp through the utility incision, mobilize the bronchus (Figure 17-8).
◆ Use the stapler through incision 3 or 4 to transect the bronchus (Figure 17-9).

Step 7. Additional Lingular Artery

◆ **Exposure:** Retract the upper lobe superiorly and apically through the utility incision.
◆ Aim the thoracoscope anteriorly and slightly medially, and point the lens toward the mediastinum and slightly posteriorly.
◆ An additional lingular artery may need to be taken, especially if the tumor is superiorly located in the lingula.
◆ With Metzenbaum scissors brought through incision 1 or 3, dissect the lingular artery.
◆ With a right-angle clamp, complete the mobilization of the artery (Figure 17-10). Use the stapler through the inferior incision to transect the artery (Figure 17-11).

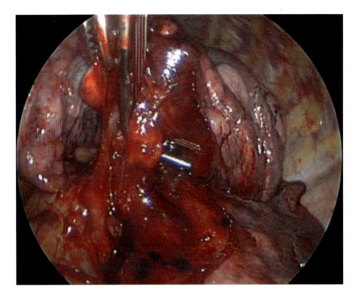

Figure 17-8. Dissection of the lingular bronchus.

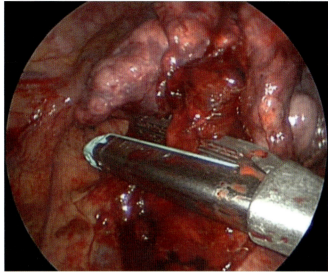

Figure 17-9. The stapler passed through the anterior incision staples the lingular bronchus.

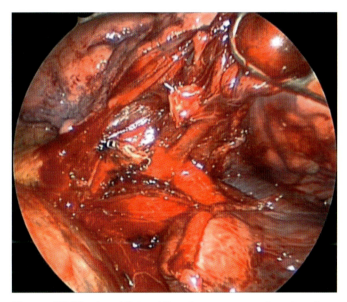

Figure 17-10. An additional lingular artery must be taken for the lingulectomy.

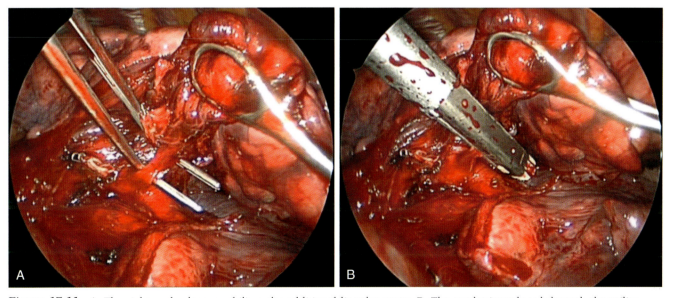

Figure 17-11. A, The right-angle clamp mobilizes the additional lingular artery. **B,** The stapler introduced through the utility incision transects the lingular artery.

Step 8. Fissure

- **Exposure:** Return the lung to its anatomic position.
- Aim the thoracoscope medially with the 30-degree lens pointed slightly posteriorly.
- There is usually a small indentation on the medial surface of the left upper lobe to mark the separation between the lingula and the upper division of the upper lobe (Figure 17-12).
- Complete the fissure with the stapler through the utility incision. The use of this incision allows the stapler to pass perpendicularly across the lobe between the lingula and the upper division. Before firing the stapler, make sure the vein and bronchus for the upper division are not compromised (Figure 17-13).

Step 9. Lingula Removal

- As described for other lobectomies (see Chapter 1), place the lingula in a bag for removal through the utility incision.

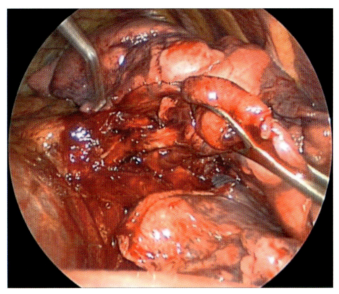

Figure 17-12. The minimal indentation between the lingula and the upper lobe helps to determine where to place the stapler to separate the lingula from the upper lobe.

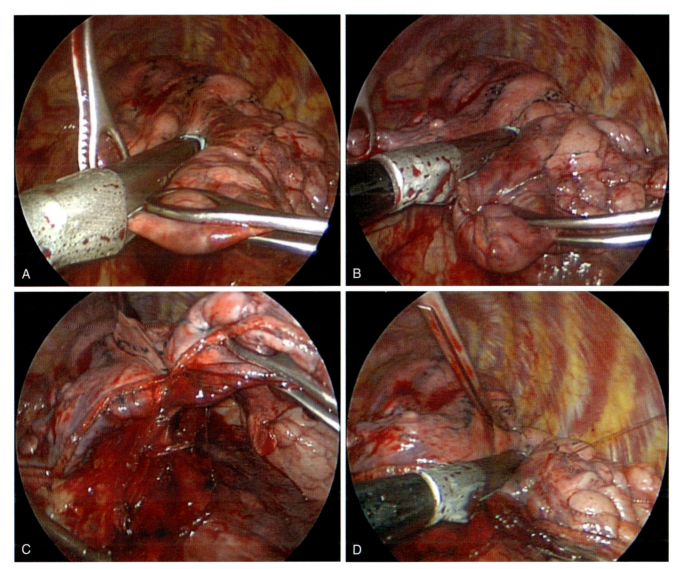

Figure 17-13. A, The stapler introduced through the anterior incision completes the fissure between the lingula and the upper division of the left upper lobe. **B-D,** Another firing of the stapler completes the fissure.

CHAPTER 18

SUPERIOR SEGMENTECTOMY—

VIDEO 18

Robert J. McKenna, Jr.

Introduction

The approach to a superior segmentectomy varies with the completeness of the fissure. If the fissure is complete, I prefer an anterior approach because the artery can be easily visualized in the fissure. If the fissure is incomplete, the entire fissure can be completed (as for a lower lobectomy [see Chapter 11]) so the anterior to posterior approach can be performed. Alternatively, the segmentectomy can be approached posteriorly.

Approach to Video-Assisted Superior Segmentectomy

Order of Operative Steps

The order of the steps for an anterior approach is as follows: major fissure, superior segmental artery, superior segmental bronchus, superior segmental vein, and the fissure. The order of the steps for a posterior approach is as follows: superior segmental bronchus, superior segmental vein, superior segmental artery, and the fissure. For a posterior approach, the order is vein, bronchus, and then artery.

Key Points

◆ Determine whether the artery can be seen in the fissure to decide which approach to take.

Anterior Approach for Superior Segmentectomy (Video 18)

Step 1. Identifying the Artery in a Major Fissure: Complete Fissure

- **Exposure:** Retract the lung directly posteriorly.
- Aim the thoracoscope anteriorly with the 30-degree lens pointed posteriorly toward the hilum.
- Use the standard incisions (see Figure 1-2 in Chapter 1).
- Elevate the lower lobe with a ring forceps introduced posteriorly, and elevate the middle lobe or upper lobe (or both) with a ring forceps introduced anteriorly. If the fissure is complete, open the pleura with Metzenbaum scissors or electrocautery through the anterior incision to identify the artery (Figure 18-1).
- Through the lower anterior incision, dissect on the surface of the artery with Metzenbaum scissors. This creates a tunnel for the stapler to complete the fissure (Figure 18-2).
- Place the anvil of the stapler on the surface of the artery; it is not moved because ring forceps anteriorly and posteriorly pull the lung parenchyma of the fissure into the stapler.
- With this approach, the artery to the superior segment is exposed (Figure 18-3).
- Directly below the fissure, continue to dissect with the Metzenbaum scissors beyond the superior segmental artery (Figure 18-4). The bronchus can be felt with the scissors. Continue this dissection through the posterior pleura to complete the remainder of the fissure.
- Place an endoscopic stapler through the anteroinferior incision to complete the fissure.

Step 2. Identifying the Artery in a Major Fissure: Incomplete Fissure

- If the fissure is very incomplete, the entire fissure can be opened with a stapler to avoid the air leaks created by dissecting in the fissure (see Chapter 11).

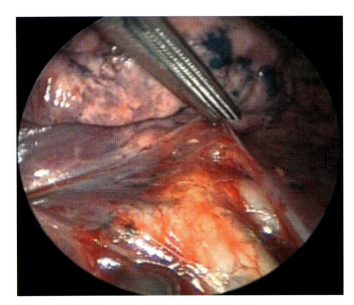

Figure 18-1. The artery is identified in the fissure.

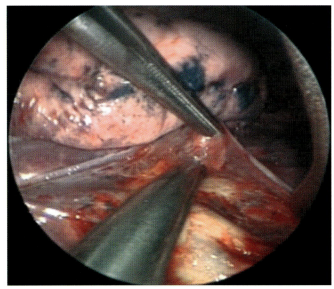

Figure 18-2. Dissection on the artery with scissors dissecting creates a tunnel for the stapler to complete the fissure.

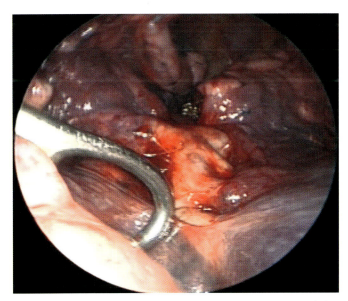

Figure 18-3. Superior segmental artery after completion of the fissure.

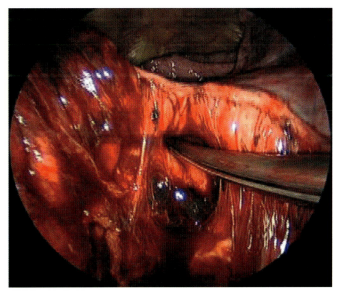

Figure 18-4. Dissection on the pulmonary artery posteriorly creates a tunnel to complete the remainder of the fissure.

Step 3. Superior Segmental Artery

◆ **Exposure:** Retract the lower lobe slightly posteriorly and inferiorly.

◆ Aim the thoracoscope anteriorly with the 30-degree lens pointed posteriorly down the fissure.

◆ Through the anterior incision, use Metzenbaum scissors and DeBakey pickups to dissect the superior segmental artery (Figure 18-5).

◆ With a vascular stapler through the anteroinferior incision, transect the superior segmental artery (Figure 18-6).

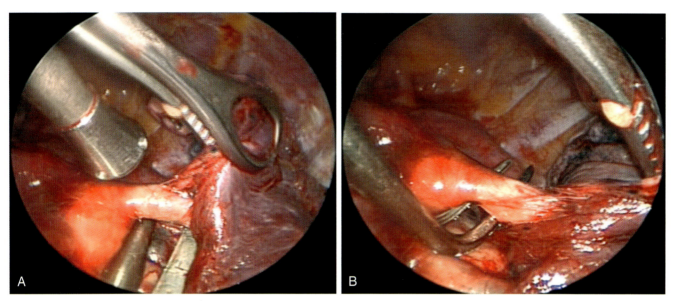

Figure 18-5. **A** and **B,** Dissection of the superior segmental artery.

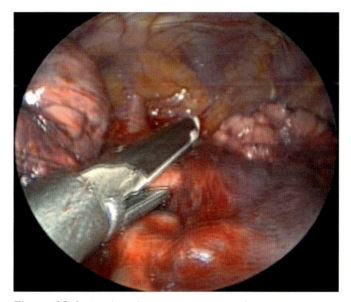

Figure 18-6. Stapling the superior segmental artery.

Step 4. Superior Segmental Bronchus

- **Exposure:** Retract the lung directly posteriorly and slightly inferiorly.
- Aim the thoracoscope anteriorly with the 30-degree lens pointed posteriorly toward the bronchus.
- If the fissure has not been completed, dissect along the superior aspect of the bronchus with the Metzenbaum scissors introduced through the inferior incision. Push with the scissors posteriorly. Except the spine, there is no significant structure posteriorly. After the tunnel is complete, staple the remainder of the fissure with a stapler through the anteroinferior incision. Place the anvil of the stapler in the tunnel and line up the cartridge with the fissure (Figure 18-7).
- Dissect the bronchus with scissors through the anterior incision.
- Transect the bronchus with a stapler through the anteroinferior incision (Figure 18-8).

Step 5. Superior Segmental Vein

- **Exposure:** Retract the lung directly posteriorly and inferiorly.
- Aim the thoracoscope anteriorly with the 30-degree lens pointed posteriorly toward the vein.
- Dissect the vein with scissors through the anterior incision.
- Transect the vein with a stapler through the anteroinferior incision.

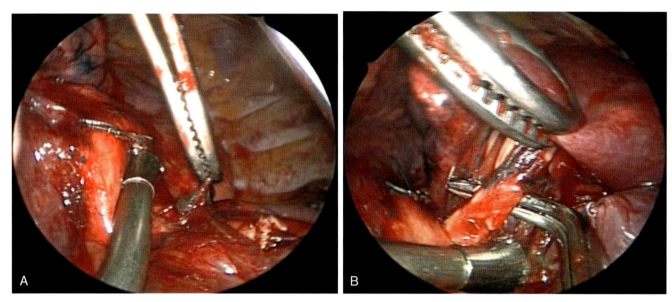

Figure 18-7. **A** and **B,** Mobilization of the superior segmental bronchus.

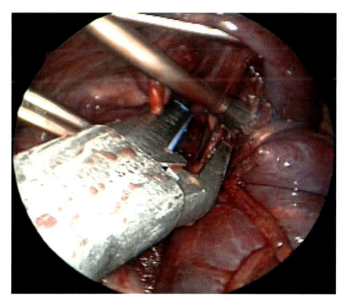

Figure 18-8. Stapling of the superior segmental bronchus.

Step 6. Separating the Superior Segment

- **Exposure:** Retract the segment superiorly.
- Aim the thoracoscope anteriorly with the 30-degree lens pointed posteriorly toward the lung.
- Pass the stapler through the anteroinferior incision. Place the anvil of the stapler just above the artery. Pull the superior segment superiorly with a ring forceps through the anterior incision (Figure 18-9).
- Occasionally, there is a small fissure between the superior segment and the basilar segments, which helps with identifying the proper location for the separation of the superior segment from the basilar segments. If not, place the stapler to provide adequate margins away from the tumor in the segment. Subsequently, place the stapler so that the anvil of the stapler is positioned in front of the artery to avoid compromising it (Figure 18-10).

Step 7. Segment Removal

- Remove the segment as described for other resections (see Chapter 1).

Posterior Approach for Superior Segmentectomy

An alternate approach for the superior segmentectomy is a posterior approach. It can be the surgeon's standard approach for a superior segmentectomy or used when there is an incomplete fissure.

- Retract the lung anteriorly.
- Dissect the vein from the superior segment, and staple it.
- Identify the bronchus found just superior to the vein. After transecting the bronchus, the artery can be seen and stapled.
- Staple the fissure.

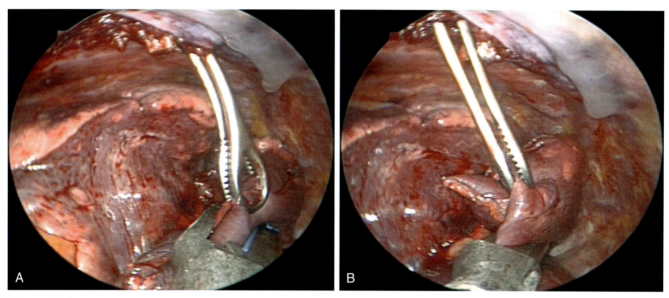

Figure 18-9. **A** and **B**, Starting to complete the fissure to separate the superior segment.

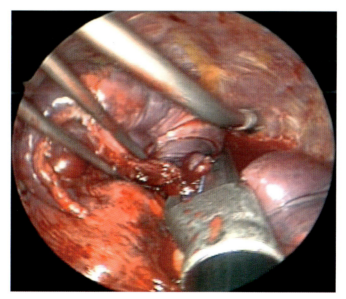

Figure 18-10. Completion of the fissure to separate the superior segment.

CHAPTER 19

RIGHT UPPER LOBE ANTERIOR SEGMENTECTOMY—VIDEO 19

Robert J. McKenna, Jr.

Introduction

This segmentectomy is infrequently performed. Many surgeons do not know how to perform it, but it is a straightforward procedure.

Approach to Video-Assisted Right Upper Lobe Anterior Segmentectomy

Order of Operative Steps
The order of the steps of the operation is as follows: minor fissure, anterior segment vein, anterior segmental artery, segmental bronchus, and the fissure.

Key Points
- Work anteriorly to posteriorly, with little manipulation of the lung.
- No posterior dissection is necessary. Very little lung manipulation is needed.

 ## Video-Assisted Right Upper Lobe Anterior Segmentectomy (Video 19)

Step 1. Incisions
- Use the standard incisions, with the utility incision placed directly up (lateral) from the superior pulmonary vein (see Figure 1-2 in Chapter 1).

Step 2. Minor Fissure

- **Exposure:** Retract the lung posteriorly and slightly inferiorly.
- Aim the thoracoscope anteriorly, and point the 30-degree lens posteriorly, but it is pulled back almost to the trocar.
- The landmarks for completion of the minor fissure are the junction of the minor and major fissures for the staple cartridge and at the confluence of the right upper lobe and right middle lobe veins for the anvil of the stapler.
- Point the anvil of the stapler toward that venous confluence. Do not move the stapler. With ring forceps, pull the lung parenchyma into the jaws of the 4.8-mm endoscopic stapler pointed toward the fissure. The first firing of the stapler usually completes about one half of the fissure.
- With the Metzenbaum scissors through the utility incision, dissect along the inferior aspect of the right upper lobe vein to expose the pulmonary artery that lies posterior and perpendicular to the vein. Dissect the surface of the artery.
- Place the anvil of the stapler between the veins and on the surface of the artery for additional firings of the stapler (Figure 19-1A). Do not move the stapler.
- Open the jaws of the stapler, and pull the lung parenchyma into the jaws of the stapler with ring forceps.
- Fire the stapler to complete the minor fissure (Figure 19-1B).

Step 3. Anterior Segmental Vein

- **Exposure:** Retract the lung directly posteriorly.
- Aim the thoracoscope anteriorly with the 30-degree lens pointed posteriorly.
- Dissect along the inferior aspect of the upper lobe vein. The inferior-most branch is the vein from the anterior segment (Figure 19-2).
- With Metzenbaum scissors through incision 3, dissect the vein, and widely spread a right-angle clamp to create a wide tunnel through which to pass the anvil of the stapler (Figure 19-3).
- Pass the vascular stapler through incision 4 (or 3) to transect the vein.

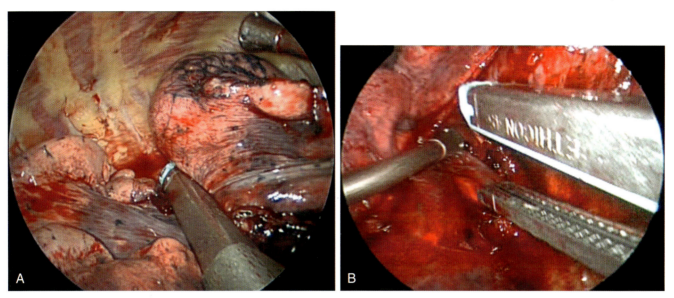

Figure 19-1. A, Positioning the cartridge of the stapler to complete the minor fissure. **B,** Positioning the anvil of the stapler to complete the minor fissure.

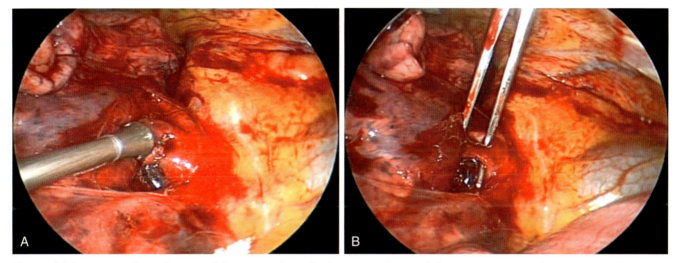

Figure 19-2. A, Veins from the upper lobe. **B,** A right-angle clamp passed around the anterior segmental vein exposes the artery behind the vein.

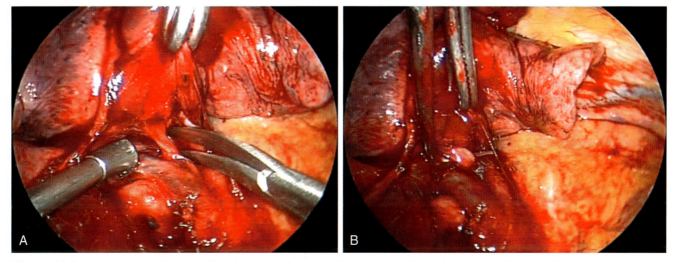

Figure 19-3. A, Scissors used to mobilize the anterior segmental artery. **B,** Right-angle clamp used to mobilize the anterior segmental artery.

Step 4. Anterior Segmental Artery

◆ **Exposure:** Retract the lung posteriorly and slightly inferiorly.
◆ Aim the thoracoscope anteriorly with the 30-degree lens pointed posteriorly. Rotate the camera slightly clockwise.
◆ The anterior segmental artery can be seen after the vein has been transected.
◆ Through incision 3, use Metzenbaum scissors to dissect the anterior segmental artery.
◆ The bronchus is directly behind the artery. Pass a right-angle clamp between the artery and the bronchus, and spread widely to create a tunnel for the stapler.
◆ Transect the artery with a vascular stapler from incision 3 or incision 4 (Figure 19-4).

Step 5. Anterior Segmental Bronchus

◆ **Exposure:** Retract the lung posteriorly and slightly superiorly.
◆ Aim the thoracoscope anteriorly with the 30-degree lens pointed posteriorly.
◆ Remove the segmental (level 12) nodes from the surface of the segmental bronchus (Figure 19-5).
◆ Dissect the anterior segmental bronchus with Metzenbaum scissors through incision 3.
◆ Behind the bronchus is a small artery that goes to the apical segment. Pass a right-angle clamp between the artery and the bronchus, and spread the clamp widely to create a tunnel for the stapler.
◆ Transect the bronchus with a stapler from incision 4 (or incision 3) (Figure 19-6).

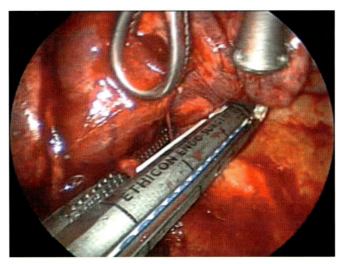

Figure 19-4. Stapler used to transect the anterior segmental artery.

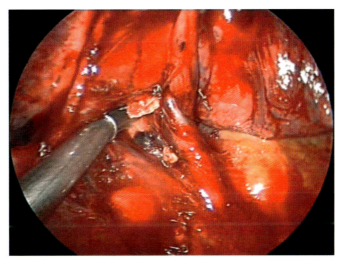

Figure 19-5. Segmental nodes on the anterior segmental bronchus.

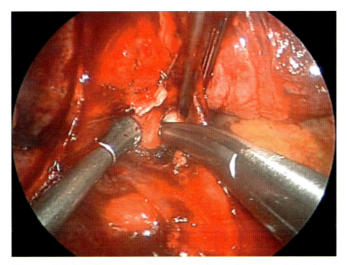

Figure 19-6. The anterior segmental bronchus is mobilized with the scissors.

Step 6. Fissure between the Anterior and Apical Segments

- **Exposure:** Retract the lung directly posteriorly and apically.
- Aim the thoracoscope anteriorly with the 30-degree lens pointed posteriorly.
- Separate the anterior segment from the apical segment with a 4.8-mm endoscopic stapler (Figure 19-7).

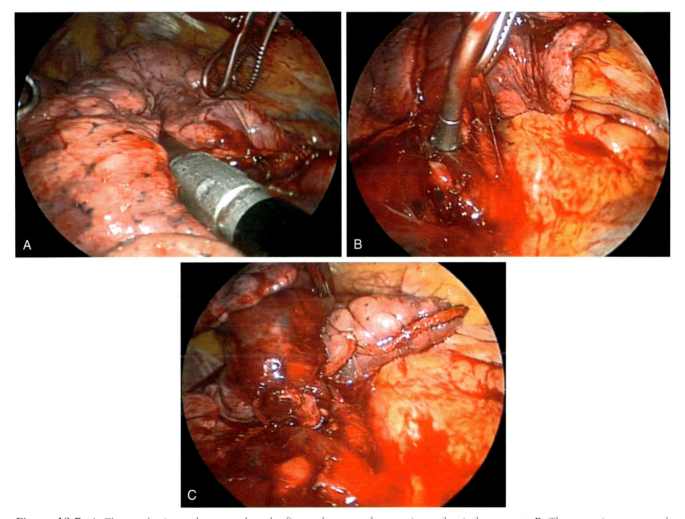

Figure 19-7. A, The stapler is used to complete the fissure between the anterior and apical segments. **B**, The posterior segmental vein should be preserved when transecting the anterior segmental artery. **C**, Completion of the fissure exposes the bronchus.

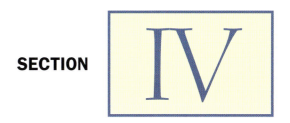

SECTION IV

Mediastinal and Esophageal Procedures

CHAPTER 20

VIDEO–ASSISTED MEDIASTINOSCOPY — VIDEO 20

Robert J. McKenna, Jr.

Introduction

Mediastinoscopy is an important staging procedure for lung cancer. Development of video-assisted mediastinoscopy has greatly improved the quality and safety of the procedure that can be performed. Node dissection can be performed with the standard video mediastinoscope.

Approach to Video-Assisted Mediastinoscopy

Order of Operative Steps

Mediastinoscopy can be performed inferiorly to superiorly or vice versa. Usually, surgeons start inferiorly, and the steps of the procedure are as follows: subcarinal nodes, pretracheal nodes, level 4 nodes, and level 2 nodes.

Key Points

- Work inferiorly to superiorly.
- Before inserting the mediastinoscope, bluntly dissect with a finger to separate matted nodes from major vessels.
- Dissect on named structures to perform a complete node dissection.
- An assistant can hold the mediastinoscope so the surgeon may use two instruments for dissection: biopsy forceps and the suction tip.

Video-Assisted Mediastinoscopy

Step 1. Incision

- Make a 2-cm incision (Figure 20-1) transversely in the base of the neck that is 1 or 2 fingerbreadths above the sternal notch.
- With electrocautery, cut transversely through the platysma muscle and then vertically in the midline between the strap muscles.
- With a closed Kelly clamp, bluntly dissect in the midline between the muscles to expose the trachea.
- Sweep the widely spread clamp along the surface of the trachea.
- Place an Army-Navy retractor between the fascia and the surface of the trachea. Lift anteriorly.
- Bluntly dissect with a finger on the surface of the trachea as far as possible into the chest.
- The finger breaks through the pretracheal fascia to mobilize the lymph nodes as much as possible. This often is the safest method to dissect matted nodes away from vessels.

Step 2. Level 7 Nodes

- Bluntly dissect the anterior surfaces of the right and left mainstem bronchi.
- An artery can usually be seen passing from the aorta to the carina. Clip the artery to reduce bleeding during removal of the subcarinal nodes (Figure 20-2).
- Bluntly dissect along the posterior aspect of the pulmonary artery.
- Dissect along the medial aspect of the left mainstem bronchus inferiorly to the carina. The blunt-tipped suction then sweeps the subcarinal nodes from left to right and off the surface of the esophagus.
- Similarly, dissect along the medial aspect of the right mainstem bronchus.
- Hold the subcarinal nodes to the right to allow blunt dissection between the nodes and the esophagus (Figure 20-3).
- Remove all the subcarinal nodes until both mainstem bronchi and the esophagus have been completely exposed (Figure 20-4).
- Place a Surgicel hemostat in the subcarinal space for hemostasis.

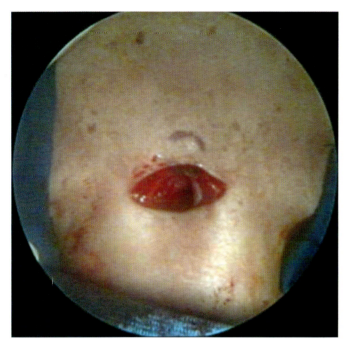

Figure 20-1. Incision for introducing the mediastinoscope.

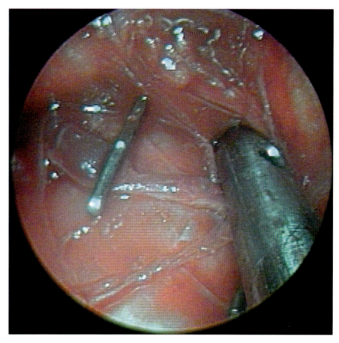

Figure 20-2. The artery travels from the aorta *(left)* to the carina. It can be clipped as shown.

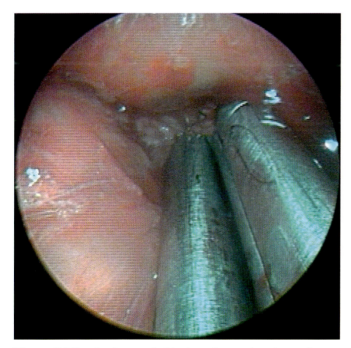

Figure 20-3. The forceps holds the subcarinal nodes to the right as the suction dissects along the medial aspect of the left mainstem bronchus.

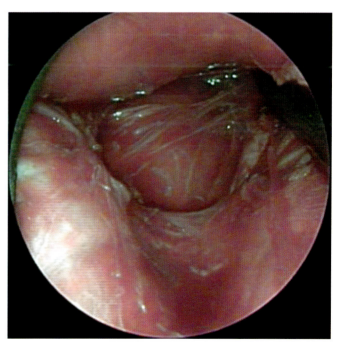

Figure 20-4. Empty subcarinal space after node dissection.

Step 3. Left Level 10 Nodes
- Bluntly dissect along the lateral aspect of the left mainstem bronchus to avoid pressure on the left recurrent laryngeal nerve, which can be seen (Figure 20-5).
- Bluntly mobilize the level 10 nodes with as little pressure on the nerve as possible.

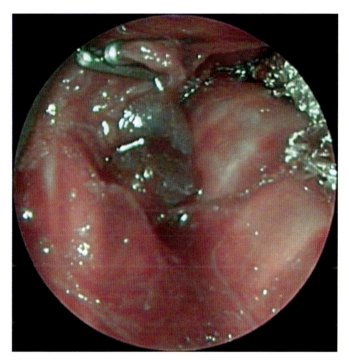

Figure 20-5. Level 10 nodes.

Step 4. Right Level 10 Nodes

◆ Bluntly dissect along the lateral aspect of the right mainstem bronchus.
◆ Laterally, dissect along the azygous vein to the superior vena cava anteriorly.
◆ Remove the right level 10 nodes along the mainstem bronchus.
◆ Dissect along the pulmonary artery in this area. The right truncus anterior often can be identified (Figure 20-6).

Step 5. Level 4 and 2 Nodes

◆ With the biopsy forceps, grasp the fatty tissue anterior to the distal trachea, and pull posteriorly away from the superior vena cava.
◆ With the suction tip, bluntly dissect horizontally to identify the superior vena cava.
◆ Remove all nodes and fatty material (Figure 20-7).

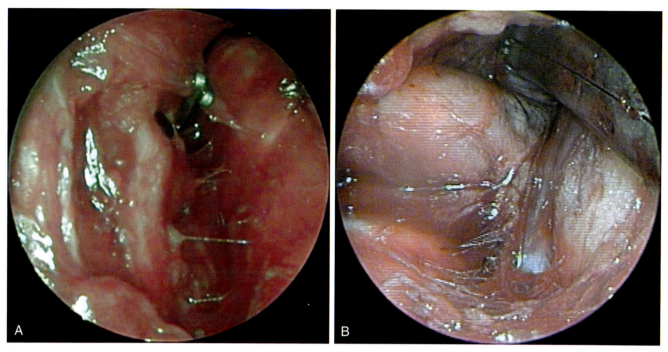

Figure 20-6. **A,** Left recurrent laryngeal nerve. **B,** Right mainstem bronchus, azygous vein, and anterior trunk.

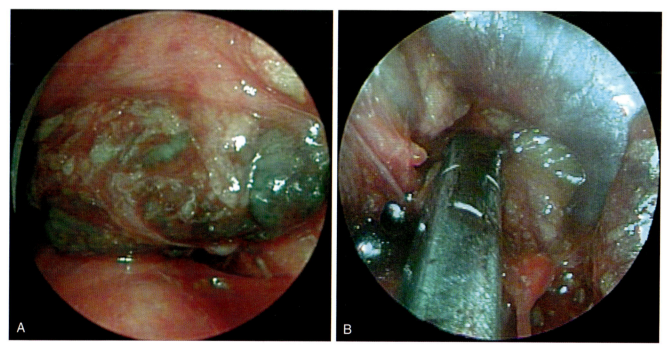

Figure 20-7. **A,** Level R4 node. **B,** Exposure of the superior vena cava and azygous vein.

- There is often a small vein from the nodes to the superior vena cava. Identify and clip the vein (Figure 20-8).
- Continue dissection until all of the tissue between the azygous vein to the innominate artery has been removed (Figures. 20-9 and 20-10).

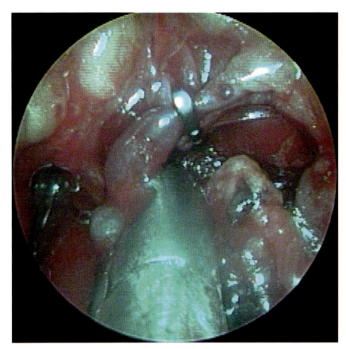

Figure 20-8. Clipped vein from the nodes to the superior vena cava.

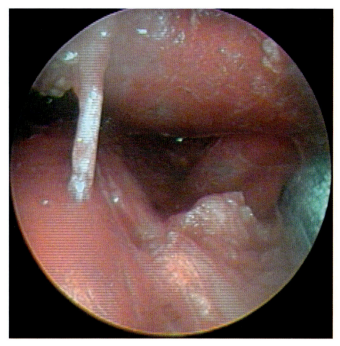

Figure 20-9. Empty space from the carina to the innominate artery.

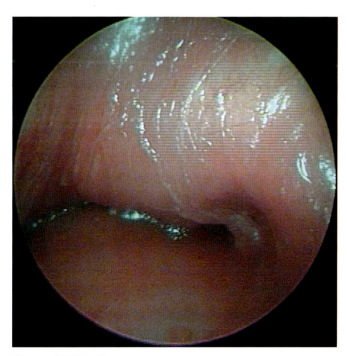

Figure 20-10. The innominate artery.

CHAPTER 21

RIGHT-SIDED MEDIASTINAL LYMPH NODE DISSECTION—VIDEO 21

Ali Mahtabifard

Introduction

Right-sided and left-sided mediastinal lymph node dissections are discussed in separate chapters. No additional incisions are made for the mediastinal lymph node dissection; the procedure uses the existing incisions for the video-assisted lobectomy, which usually precedes the dissection.

Approach to Video-Assisted Right-Sided Mediastinal Lymph Node Dissection

Order of Operative Steps

The order of the steps of the lymph node dissection is as follows: level 9 and 8 nodes, level 7 nodes, level 10 nodes, and level 4 and 2 nodes.

Key Points

- Subcarinal lymph node dissection usually is easier on the right side.
- Transection of the azygous vein can simplify the level 2 and 4 node dissection.
- Use of electrocautery near nerves should be kept to a minimum. Nuisance bleeding from the lymph node dissection bed usually can be controlled with pressure or a Surgicel.

 ## Video-Assisted Right-Sided Mediastinal Lymph Node Dissection

Step 1. Level 9 and 8 Lymph Nodes

- **Exposure:** Hold the right lower lobe superiorly with a ring clamp through the utility incision.
- Aim the thoracoscope anteriorly, and point the 30-degree lens downward toward the inferior pulmonary ligament.

- Bring the suction catheter and the long-tipped electrocautery through the anteroinferior incision. Press the curve of the Yankauer suction catheter onto the diaphragm to hold it out of the way.
- If the diaphragm is high and in the way, as is seen frequently in obese patients, place a heavy stitch in the ligamentous portion of the diaphragm. Pull the stitch through the incision for the trocar. Suture it to the skin to retract the diaphragm.
- Hold the inferior pulmonary ligament toward the apex of the chest. Level 9 lymph nodes can be seen.
- Incise the inferior pulmonary ligament with the long-tipped electrocautery up to the level of the inferior pulmonary vein as shown in Figure 21-1. The tip of the suction catheter should be held close to the electrocautery tip to remove the smoke created.
- Remove the level 9 lymph nodes as the ligament is incised.

Step 2. Level 7 Lymph Nodes

- **Exposure:** Hold the right lower lobe superiorly with a ring clamp through the utility incision.
- Aim the thoracoscope anteriorly, and point the 30-degree lens downward toward the inferior pulmonary ligament.
- With ring forceps, which are brought through the inferior and the utility incisions, retract the right lower lobe medially toward the heart.
- Point the thoracoscope posteriorly and the 30-degree lens toward the esophagus.
- Incise the posterior mediastinal pleura with scissors, which are brought through the anterior incision as shown in Figure 21-2. Carefully incise the pleura at its junction with the lung parenchyma. The natural tendency is to gravitate posteriorly toward the esophagus, but this should be avoided because it causes nuisance bleeding from the esophageal muscle.
- In the process of this dissection, remove the paraesophageal level 8 lymph nodes.
- Multiple instruments can be brought through each incision. Remove lymph nodes through the utility incision. If lymph nodes containing metastases are pulled through a small incision, cancer cells may be squeezed into the tissues, and the cancer may recur in the incisions.
- At this point, the inferior pulmonary vein and the posterior aspect of the bronchus intermedius are evident.
- Dissect the border of the bronchus intermedius, which ultimately leads to the subcarinal lymph node station. A combination of sharp and blunt dissection is used to reach station 7 and to remove the nodes as demonstrated in Video 21-1. The dissection planes include the esophagus posteriorly, the pericardium anteriorly, and the carina superiorly.
- Clip or cauterize the bronchial artery that is usually found at the carina.
- After complete lymphadenectomy of the subcarinal region, the right and left mainstem bronchi are visualized (Figure 21-3).
- Place a folded Surgicel in the subcarinal region to tamponade any oozing.

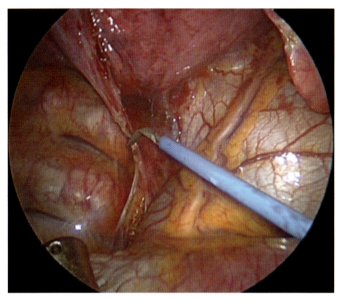

Figure 21-1. The inferior pulmonary ligament is on stretch and is cauterized through the anteroinferior incision.

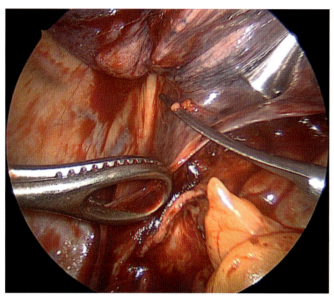

Figure 21-2. Posterior aspects of the inferior pulmonary vein and the bronchus intermedius.

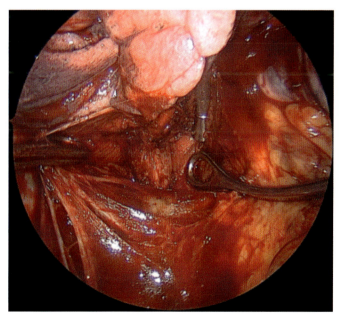

Figure 21-3. The posterior mediastinal pleura is incised at its junction with the lung parenchyma. The scissors are brought through the anterior incision.

Step 3. Level 10 Lymph Nodes

- **Exposure:** Pull the right upper lobe (if a prior right upper lobectomy has not been performed) with a long, curved ring clamp inferiorly and posteriorly. If a right upper lobectomy has been performed, with a ring clamp through the anteroinferior incision, pull the middle and the lower lobes posteriorly. With this exposure, dissect the 10, 4, 2, and 3 lymph node stations through the utility incision.
- Aim the thoracoscope anteriorly, and point the 30-degree lens at the superior hilar region.
- Identify the triangle, which is bordered by the superior aspect of the right hilum, the azygous vein, and the superior vena cava (SVC) (Figure 21-4).
- With the Metzenbaum scissors brought through the anterior incision, incise the pleura along these named structures to begin the nodal dissection.
- Remove all the soft tissue in this level 10 station with a combination of sharp dissection using the scissors and blunt dissection using the suction catheter.
- Remove all tissue and lymph nodes through the utility incision in case they contain cancer cells.
- Sharply dissect posteriorly on the surface of the vein from the apex of the right upper lobe as it passes over the superior hilum. This exposes the anterior trunk of the right pulmonary artery. After these lymph nodes are removed (Figure 21-5), bluntly dissect between the anterior trunk and the right mainstem bronchus if the right upper lobe is to be resected.

Step 4. Level 4 and 2 Lymph Nodes

- **Exposure:** The exposure is not changed.
- The position of the thoracoscope is not changed.
- Incise the mediastinal pleura on the superior aspect of the azygous vein and parallel to the SVC. Identify the phrenic nerve on the lateral aspect of the SVC (Figure 21-6). To avoid damaging the nerve, turn the scissors tips so the phrenic nerve can be seen (Figure 21-7).

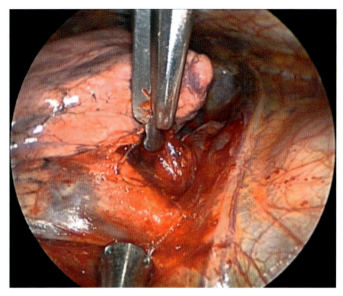

Figure 21-4. Station 10 lymph nodes are found in the triangle bordered by the superior aspect of the right hilum, the azygous vein, and the superior vena cava. Removal of these lymph nodes facilitates subsequent isolation of the anterior trunk for a right upper lobectomy.

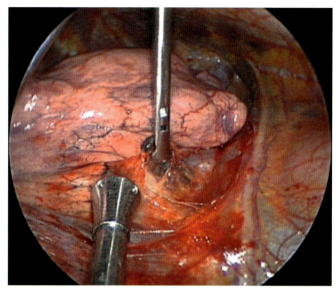

Figure 21-5. Removal of lobar lymph nodes in this region helps to expose the pulmonary artery branches.

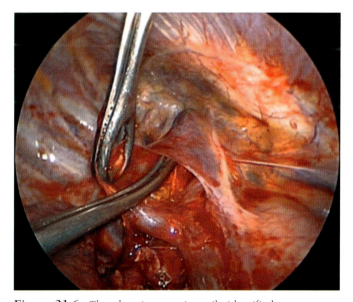

Figure 21-6. The phrenic nerve is easily identified.

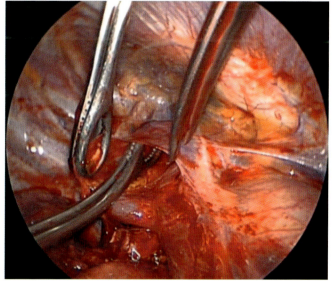

Figure 21-7. The mediastinal pleura is incised while visualizing both tips of the Metzenbaum scissors and the phrenic nerve.

- Isolate the azygous vein with the right-angle clamp, which is brought through the utility incision (Figure 21-8).
- Bring a vascular stapler through the posterior incision to transect the azygous vein (Figure 21-9).
- With a combination of blunt and sharp dissection, remove all the tissue between the SVC, the pericardium over the ascending aorta, and trachea from the level of the pulmonary artery to the innominate artery. This removes all level 4 and 2 lymph nodes. Visualize but do not cut the vagus nerve posteriorly (Figure 21-10).
- Grasp the lymph node packet in each station with a ring clamp, which can be brought through the utility incision or through the posterior incision. Hold the tissue posteriorly and away from the SVC (Figure 21-11). Use electrocautery for the dissection to minimize bleeding.

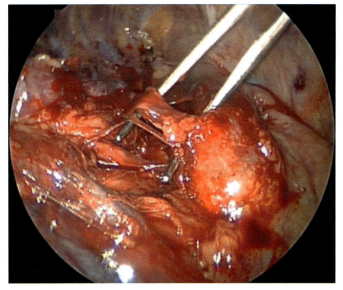

Figure 21-8. The azygous vein is isolated with a right-angle clamp.

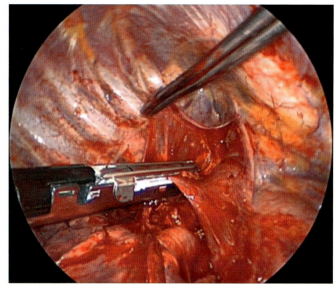

Figure 21-9. The azygous vein is transected with a vascular stapler through the posterior incision. This step facilitates level 4 lymph node dissection.

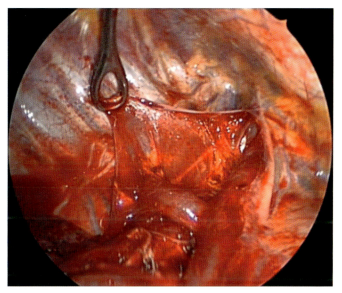

Figure 21-10. The vagus nerve must be avoided.

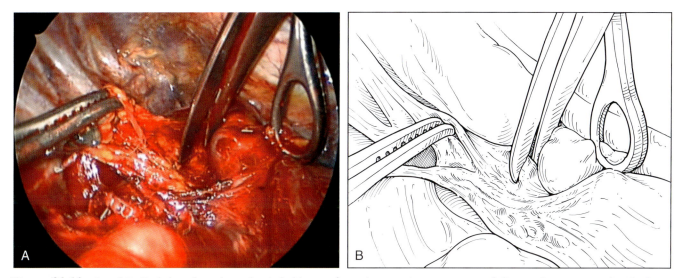

Figure 21-11. A and **B**, Each lymph node packet is held away from the superior vena cava and dissected or transected with the scissors or electrocautery. Electrocautery in this region must be used with great care.

- Often, a small vein drains the level 4 nodes into the SVC. It should be identified and clipped (Figure 21-12).
- Continue this process in a cephalad direction to dissect the level 3 and 2 lymph nodes (Figure 21-13).
- A complete mediastinal lymph node dissection done with video-assisted thoracic surgery (VATS) often provides better visualization than with a thoracotomy.
- On completion of the full lymph node dissection, the paratracheal region is bare, and the important anatomic landmarks are clearly identified (Figure 21-14).
- Minimize usage of electrocautery at the superior margin of this dissection to prevent damage to the recurrent laryngeal nerve. A Surgicel can be tucked into this space for improved hemostasis (Figure 21-15).

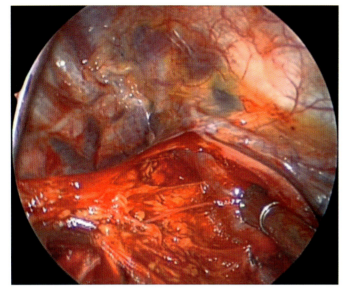

Figure 21-12. Occasionally, a small vein draining level 4 lymph nodes into the superior vena cava is identified. It is best clipped and cut.

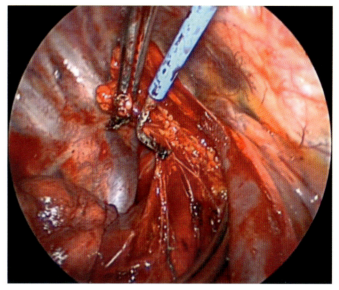

Figure 21-13. The dissection continues in a cephalad direction to include levels 3 and 2.

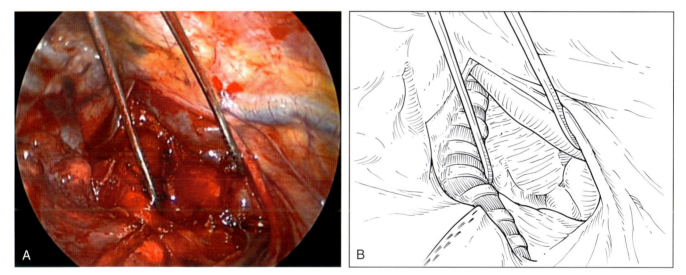

Figure 21-14. **A** and **B**, Important anatomic landmarks are shown after completion of a thorough lymph node dissection.

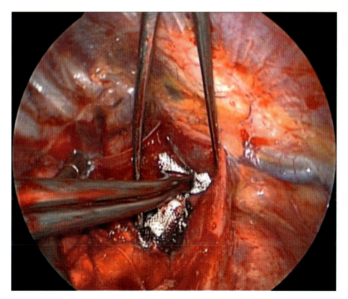

Figure 21-15. A Surgicel placed in the bed of the dissected lymph node stations ensures hemostasis.

CHAPTER 22

LEFT-SIDED MEDIASTINAL LYMPH NODE DISSECTION — VIDEO 22

Seth D. Force

Introduction

Mediastinal lymph node dissection is a critical part of any lung cancer operation. Lymph node dissection should be performed for all types of cancer resections (e.g., wedge, segmentectomy, lobectomy, pneumonectomy) to ensure proper tumor staging and for possible therapeutic benefit. Nodal dissection for left-sided resections should include station 5 (subaortic, between the aorta and left main pulmonary artery), station 6 (para-aortic, left side of the ascending aorta, and aortic arch), station 7 (subcarinal), station 8 (para-esophageal), and station 9L (inferior pulmonary vein). Video-assisted thoracic surgery (VATS) provides excellent visualization of the aortopulmonary window lymph nodes and has replaced anterior mediastinotomy (i.e., Chamberlain procedure) for biopsying nodes in this area at many institutions.

Approach to Video-Assisted Left-Sided Mediastinal Lymph Node Dissection

Order of Operative Steps

The lymph node dissection for right- and left-sided lung cancers can be performed after the parenchymal resection or can be performed before the resection, because node dissection can define the anatomy and make the lobectomy easier and because node dissection may identify stage III patients who would then undergo neoadjuvant treatment and lobectomy at another time. Exceptions include nodes in station 9, which are removed when the inferior pulmonary ligament is divided, and lymph nodes in station 10, which are usually dissected and removed just before division of the bronchus. Station 10 lymph nodes are not considered to be mediastinal nodes in the American lymph node mapping system, but they are mentioned here because unlike other N1 nodes, a standard lobectomy without a dedicated lymph node dissection may miss these nodes.

Key Points

- Carry out lymph node dissection through the standard VATS port sites using a 5- or 10-mm, 30-degree thoracoscope (Figure 22-1).
- With small ringed forceps, grasp the lymph nodes, which are friable and tend to disintegrate if only parts of them are grabbed. Alternatively, use a long Allis clamp to grasp the lymph nodes during the dissection.
- Dissect with standard electrocautery or an ultrasonic dissector. A partially covered Teflon-coated electrocautery can be used to avoid injury to surrounding structures. In some areas, adjacent structures may be at risk for injury during lymph node removal:
  - ▲ Station 7, the esophagus and mainstem bronchus: The vagus nerve should be left with the esophagus and can be used as a posterior landmark when dissecting in the level 7 area.
  - ▲ Station 9: To avoid esophageal injury during division of the inferior pulmonary ligament, keep the dissection close to the lung parenchyma. The inferior pulmonary vein is also at risk for injury during this dissection.
  - ▲ Stations 5 and 6: The left recurrent laryngeal nerve, left phrenic nerve, left main pulmonary artery, and aorta should be avoided.
- Bleeding from torn lymph nodes and bronchial arteries should be controlled with precise visualization and electrocautery. The errant use of "scorched earth" electrocautery is ill advised and is likely to lead to injury of adjacent structures. A small amount of surgical cellulose can be used to tamponade the bleeding, which promotes hemostasis and permits better visualization and control of any nodal vessels.
- Perform a complete lymph node dissection on all patients, and resist terminating the dissection when metastases are identified in one area.

 Video-Assisted Left-Sided Mediastinal Lymph Node Dissection (Video 22)

Step 1. Station 9 Nodes

- **Exposure:** The lung is retracted superiorly.
- Aim the thoracoscope posteriorly with the 30-degree lens pointed medially toward the ligament.
- Left-sided nodal stations 5, 6, 7, and 9 are included in the dissection.
- Remove station 9 lymph nodes while dividing the inferior pulmonary ligament.
- Retract the left lower lobe cephalad through the access incision or posterior port (Figure 22-2). A ringed forceps placed alongside the camera (through the same port) pushes the diaphragm down if it is impairing visualization of the pulmonary ligament.
- Divide the inferior pulmonary ligament with electrocautery through the access incision or inferior port (Figure 22-3).
- Station 9 lymph nodes become apparent as the ligament is divided and include nodes adjacent to the inferior pulmonary vein (Figure 22-4).
- The dissection is performed close to the lymph nodes to avoid injury to the esophagus and inferior pulmonary vein.
- During a left lower lobectomy, dissect bluntly along the inferior pulmonary vein to sweep the nodes toward the lung parenchyma and leave them adherent to portion of the vein that is being removed.

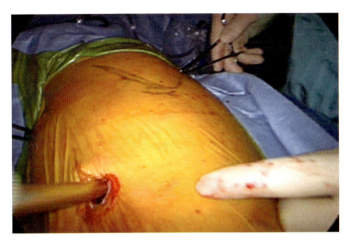

Figure 22-1. Port site placement.

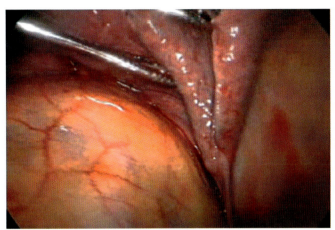

Figure 22-2. Retraction of the left lower lobe superiorly.

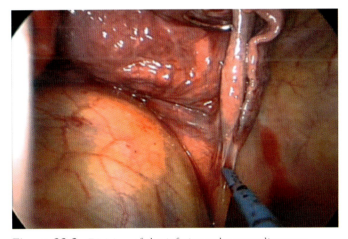

Figure 22-3. Division of the inferior pulmonary ligament.

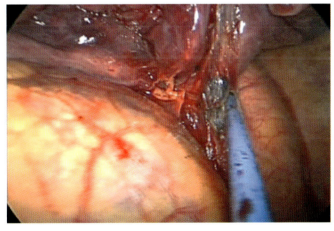

Figure 22-4. Left station 9 lymph nodes.

Step 2. Station 5 and 6 Nodes

- **Exposure:** The lung is retracted inferiorly and posteriorly.
- Aim the thoracoscope inferiorly with the 30-degree lens pointed anterior and slightly down.
- The lymph node dissection for stations 5 and 6 may be performed after the lung resection. Alternatively, resection before the lobectomy can expose and define the anatomy of the vessels and facilitate the dissection of the vessels for the lobectomy (see Chapter 11).
- Station 5 lymph nodes are located in the subaortic space between the aorta and the left main pulmonary artery.
- Station 6 lymph nodes are the para-aortic lymph nodes and are located on the left side of the ascending aorta and aortic arch.
- Occasionally, large station 5 and 6 lymph nodes obscure the view of the left upper lobe pulmonary arterial branches and require removal during the parenchymal resection.
- Retract the lung inferiorly through the posterior port, and perform the dissection through the access incision.
- Grasp the edge of the pleura, near the left main pulmonary artery, and dissect the underlying lymph nodes away from the soft tissue for removal (Figure 22-5).
- Dissect close to the nodes to avoid injury to the phrenic nerve, recurrent laryngeal nerve, and the left main pulmonary artery.
- Remove the lymph nodes through the access incision with a small ringed forceps (Figure 22-6).

Step 3. Station 7 and 10 Nodes

- **Exposure:** Retract the lung anteriorly.
- Aim the thoracoscope inferiorly with the 30-degree lens positioned posteriorly and down.
- Through the posterior port site, access the station 7 lymph nodes in the subcarinal space.
- Gently retract the aorta and esophagus posteriorly with an endokittner placed through the posterior port to open up the subcarinal space.
- Grasp the lung through the anterior access incision and retract it anteriorly (Figure 22-7).
- With electrocautery, open the pleura on the posterior hilum along the inferior border of the left lower lobe bronchus and left main bronchus.
- Place a second ringed forceps through the access incision to retract the left main bronchus anteriorly.
- Visualize the station 7 lymph nodes in the subcarinal space between the aorta and the left main bronchus (Figure 22-8).
- Grasp the nodes with a ringed forceps through the access incision or posterior port, and divide the surrounding soft tissue attachments with electrocautery.
- Locate the station 10 lymph nodes at the tracheal-bronchial angle and along the main bronchus. Remove these lymph nodes from a posterior approach during the station 7 lymph node dissection.

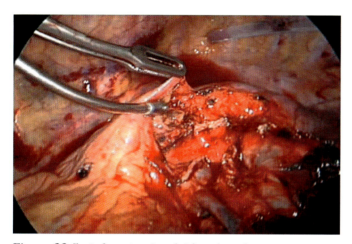

Figure 22-5. Left station 5 and 6 lymph nodes.

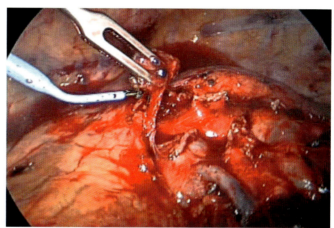

Figure 22-6. Removal of station 5 and 6 lymph nodes.

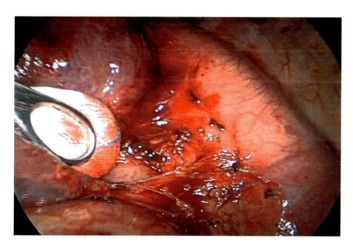

Figure 22-7. Left lung is retracted anteriorly to expose the posterior hilum and subcarinal space.

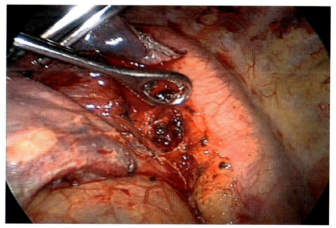

Figure 22-8. Station 7 lymph node removal.

CHAPTER 23

VIDEO-ASSISTED ESOPHAGEAL MOBILIZATION—VIDEO 23

Robert J. McKenna, Jr.

Introduction

Mobilization of the esophagus by video-assisted thoracic surgery (VATS) offers the advantage of a complete cancer operation performed with minimally invasive surgery. Although most VATS procedures are performed with the patient in the lateral decubitus position, the prone position offers several advantages for surgery on structures in the posterior mediastinum. Because gravity causes the lung to fall out of the way, lung retraction required in the lateral position is not needed when the patient is prone. Only three small incisions are needed to perform the procedure. The planes of dissection are the azygous vein, aorta, pericardium, vertebral bodies, and the trachea, allowing a thorough cancer operation with wide dissection and a complete nodal dissection to be performed.

Approach to Video-Assisted Esophageal Mobilization

Order of Operative Steps

The order of the steps of the operation are as follows: dissect on pericardium, dissect along azygous vein and aorta, remove subcarinal nodes, clip the thoracic duct, transect the azygous vein, and dissect the esophagus at the apex of the chest.

Key Points

- Perform esophagogastroduodenoscopy with the patient in the supine position on the gurney, and then place the patient prone on the operating table.
- Dissect inferiorly to superiorly in the chest.
- Dissect along the pericardium first, because if dissection along the azygous is done first, the esophagus falls in the way when dissecting the pericardial plane after the posterior dissection.

Video-Assisted Esophageal Mobilization (Video 23)

Step 1. Esophagoscopy and Positioning

- With the patient asleep and in the supine position on the gurney, perform esophago-gastroduodenoscopy.
- Move the patient in the prone position on the operating room table. Place a roll vertically under the sternum to lift the patient off the operating room table so skin preparation can include the entire posterior chest. On the right side, the preparation extends anterior to the anterior axillary line.

Step 2. Incisions

- Incision 1: Place a 5-mm trocar in the mid-axillary line in the fifth intercostal space. This is primarily used for the thoracoscope.
- Incision 2: Make a 1-cm incision in the seventh intercostal space in the posterior line.
- Incision 3: Make a 5-mm incision in the posterior axillary line in the third intercostal space.
- Encourage lung decompression with carbon dioxide insufflation.

Step 3. Anterior Esophageal Dissection

- **Exposure:** Gravity makes the lung fall anteriorly, out of the way.
- Aim the thoracoscope inferiorly with the lens pointed toward the ligament.
- Pass the thoracoscope through incision 3.
- Through incision 2, pass the Harmonic scalpel or electrocautery to cut the inferior pulmonary ligament as a grasper pulls the ligament anteriorly and superiorly.
- Dissect along the pericardium, the bronchus intermedius, and the left mainstem bronchus. This mobilizes the subcarinal lymph nodes, which are sent as a separate specimen for analysis.
- Lift the esophagus with a grasper through incision 1 (Figure 23-1).

Step 4. Posterior Esophageal Dissection

- **Exposure:** Lift the esophagus away from the azygous vein.
- Aim the thoracoscope inferiorly with the 30-degree lens pointed posteriorly.
- With the Harmonic scalpel through incision 2, mobilize the esophagus from the azygous vein.
- The esophagus is then allowed to drop anteriorly, and the aorta can be seen. Continue dissecting along the surface of the aorta. Identify small arterial branches from the aorta to the esophagus, and clip or seal them with the Harmonic scalpel. The midportion of the esophagus is completely mobilized; continue the dissection toward the diaphragm.
- Dissect the pleura by the distal esophagus parallel to the diaphragm. Clip the thoracic duct with a large endoscopic clip passed through incision 2 (Figure 23-2).
- With an endoscopic clip applier through incision 2, clip all the tissue on the lateral surface of the esophagus parallel to the diaphragm (Figure 23-3).

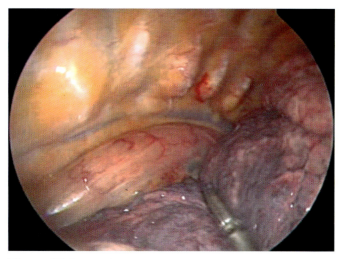

Figure 23-1. Initial exposure of the esophagus with the patient prone.

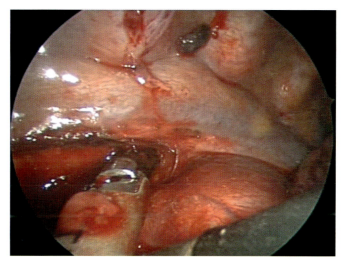

Figure 23-2. Dissection of the anterior surface of the esophagus.

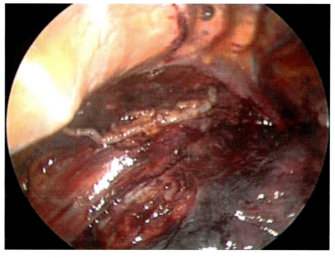

Figure 23-3. Thoracic duct for clipping.

Step 5. Dissection of the Proximal Esophagus
- **Exposure:** The lung falls anteriorly.
- Aim the thoracoscope posteriorly with the 30-degree lens pointed superiorly.
- With the Harmonic scalpel, mobilize the azygous vein as it courses anteriorly toward the superior vena cava. When it is fully mobilized, transect the azygous vein with a stapler from incision 2 (Figure 23-4).
- With a grasper through incision 3, elevate the esophagus from the posterior wall of the trachea so the Harmonic scalpel can incise the pleura and the remainder of the anterior aspect of the esophagus (Figure 23-5).
- With the grasper, pull the esophagus away from the spine so the Harmonic scalpel can incise the pleura and the rest of the esophagus from the spine. This dissection can be carried into the neck (Figure 23-6).

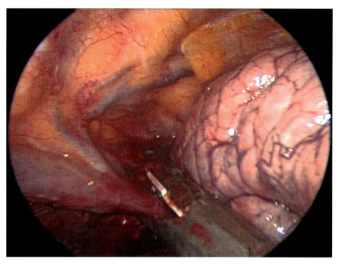

Figure 23-4. Stapler across the azygous vein.

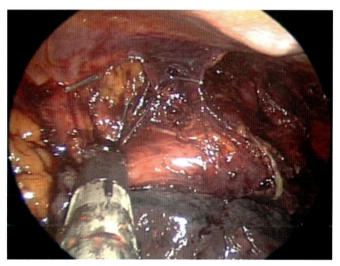

Figure 23-5. Clipping the tissue on the lateral surface of the esophagus near the diaphragm.

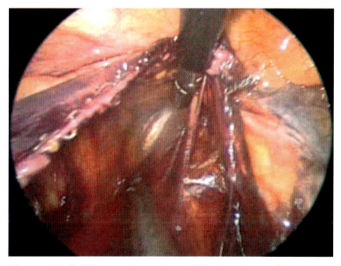

Figure 23-6. The esophagus is mobilized to the neck.

CHAPTER 24

ROBOT–ASSISTED, TWO–STAGE, THREE–FIELD ESOPHAGOLYMPHADENECTOMY— VIDEO 24

James T. Wu and Kemp H. Kernstine

Introduction

The da Vinci S system has three components: an operating console for the surgeon; a praying mantis–like chassis from which spring the robotic video unit and the three robotic arms; and the electronic communication tower system between the console and the chassis (Figure 24-1).

Approach to Robot-Assisted Esophagolymphadenectomy

Order of Operative Steps

The order of the steps of the operation are as follows: in the thoracic phase, patient positioning, port placement, docking, en bloc esophageal mobilization and wide nodal resection, cervical lymphadenectomy, thoracic duct ligation, and drain placement; then isolation of the cervical esophagus; in the abdominal phase, patient positioning, port placement, docking, placement of a feeding jejunostomy, celiac axis lymphadenectomy, and creation of a gastric conduit; and esophagogastric anastomosis.

Key Points

- A thoracotomy tray should be in the operating room at all times.
- A ring clamp with a heavy sponge or Surgicel attached should be available for immediate use at all times (Figure 24-2).
- Use continuous intrathoracic carbon dioxide insufflation to enhance the robot-assisted surgery. Keep the intrathoracic carbon dioxide pressure between 10 and 15 mm Hg to minimize a decrease in venous return and cardiac compliance.
- Small lymphatic tributaries seen under high robotic magnification are endoclipped through the accessory port or robotically.

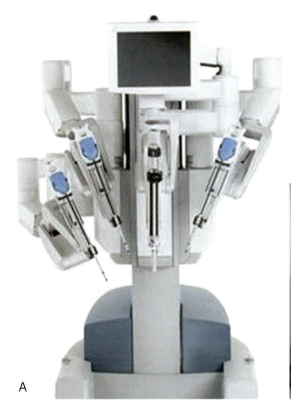

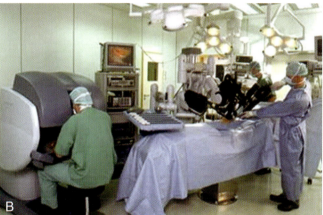

Figure 24-1. A, Intuitive Surgical's da Vinci system. **B,** Typical operating room setup.

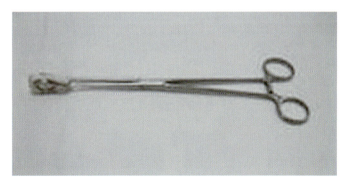

Figure 24-2. Ring clamp with attached Surgicel.

Robot-Assisted Esophagolymphadenectomy (Video 24)

Step 1. Thoracic-Phase Patient Positioning

- The patient is intubated with a double-lumen endotracheal tube, positioned laterally to slightly face down, and strapped securely to the operating table.
- The right arm is well padded and positioned over the ear immediately adjacent to the face with the elbow below the horizontal plane of the right shoulder.
- Tilt the operating table as far anteriorly as possible so that the patient is positioned 30 to 45 degrees from prone (Figure 24-3).

Step 2. Thoracic-Phase Port Placement

- Make five puncture wounds in the right mid-anterolateral chest. Place a 12-mm trocar for the viewing port in the fifth or sixth intercostal space in the posterior axillary line. Place an 8-mm trocar for the right robotic arm in the posterior axillary line just anterior to the border of the scapula in the third or fourth intercostal space. Place an additional 8-mm trocar for the left robotic arm in the seventh or eighth intercostal space in the posterior axillary line, each of the two robotic arms approximately one hand bredth away from the videoscope port (Figure 24-4).
- Place two accessory ports at the level of the anterior axillary line: a 5-mm port at the level of the third intercostal space and a 12-mm port at the level of the sixth or seventh intercostal space. The upper port is used for suctioning and grasping instruments, and the lower port is used for placing a fan retractor for the lung, suctioning and grasping instruments, and introducing the sutures used for the thoracic duct ligation.

Step 3. Thoracic-Phase Docking

- Roll the robot into position. Place the robotic arms through the 8-mm trocars, and place the 0-degree videoscope through the 12-mm viewing port (Figure 24-5).
- Carbon dioxide is insufflated to a pressure of 10 mm Hg to evacuate electrocautery smoke and to compress the lung away from the surgical site.

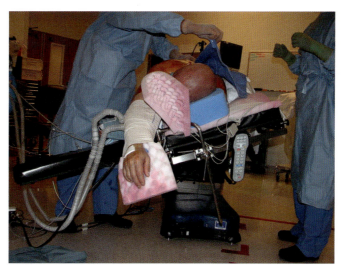

Figure 24-3. The patient is intubated with a double-lumen endotracheal tube, and the body is positioned in the left lateral decubitus position and slightly forward.

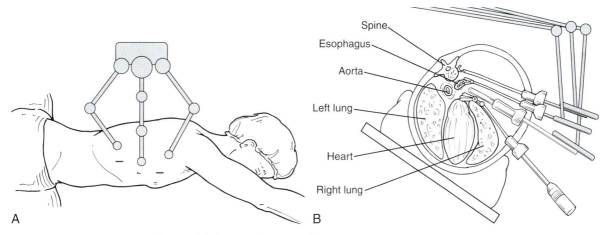

A   B

Figure 24-4. **A** and **B**, Port placement in the thoracic phase.

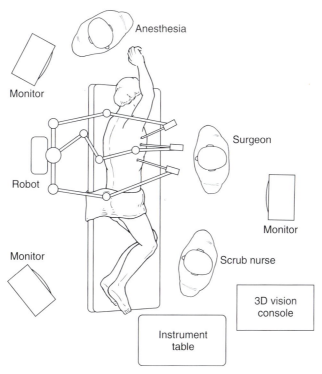

Figure 24-5. Positioning of the patient after docking.

Step 4. En Bloc Esophageal Mobilization and Wide Nodal Resection

* **Exposure:** Direct the camera toward the pericardial bulge just cephalad to the inferior pulmonary vein.
* Set the videoscope in a 0-degree position.
* Using the hook electrocautery, and/or ultrasonic shears, and Caudier grasper (Intuitive Surgical, Sunnyvale, Calif), initiate dissection along the anterior aspect of the esophagus at the pericardial bulge, just cephalad to the superior aspect of the inferior pulmonary vein (Figure 24-6).
* Continue the dissection inferiorly to the esophageal hiatus, with the inferior pulmonary ligament and adherent lung taken down as necessary for access to the periesophageal nodes, completely cleaning the pericardium, hiatus, and left pleura (Figure 24-7).
* Clear both hila of nodal tissue, and take them contiguously with the specimen (Figure 24-8).
* Take the periaortic-spinal-azygous nodes and if necessary the thoracic duct en bloc.
* Continue the dissection along the azygous vein, which is preserved when the vein is uninvolved.

Step 5. Cervical Lymphadenectomy

* **Exposure:** Direct the camera toward the thoracic inlet.
* Set the videoscope in the 0-degree position.
* Resect the supra-azygous esophagus and periesophageal tissue into the thoracic apex, well into the neck. Over the intended resection area, score the pleura with the hook electrocautery. Transect the associated peritracheal nodes and the right vagus nerve with the ultrasonic shears, reducing the potential of electrical transmission to the recurrent laryngeal nerve.
* Completely clean the posterior and rightward aspect of the trachea and the thoracic peritracheal and cervical spaces of periesophageal tissue, and continue the dissection into the thoracic inlet to the level of the inferior laryngeal cartilage (Figure 24-9).

Step 6. Thoracic Duct Ligation

* **Exposure:** Direct the camera toward the esophageal hiatus.
* Set the videoscope in a 0-degree down position.
* At the level of the diaphragm, the thoracic duct is triply ligated with 2-0 Ethibond suture, cut to an 8-cm length, encompassing all of the tissue between the azygous vein and the aorta.

Step 7. Drain Placement

* At the conclusion of the thoracic phase, place two drains: a 19-French, round, fluted Silastic drain (Blake, Ethicon Incorporated, Johnson & Johnson) through the lower accessory trocar along the diaphragm and a 15-French drain to the superior aspect of the thoracic cavity through the upper accessory trocar (Figure 24-10).
* Remove the robotic arms, and move the robot away from the patient.
* Close the thoracic trocar sites with 3-0 Vicryl sutures with an SH needle.

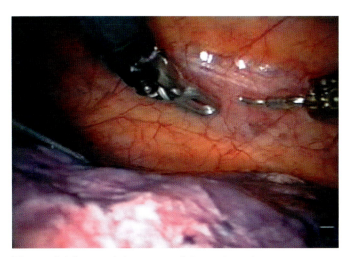

Figure 24-6. Initial dissection of the mid-esophagus.

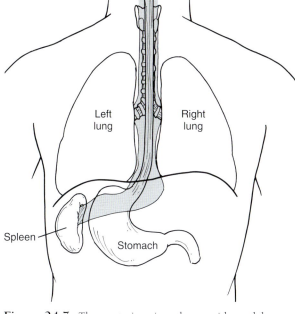

Figure 24-7. The posterior view shows wide nodal resection performed en bloc with the esophagus. The *shaded area* represents the intended borders of the resection. The surgical goal was wide and continuous resection of all of the periesophageal lymphatic tissue.

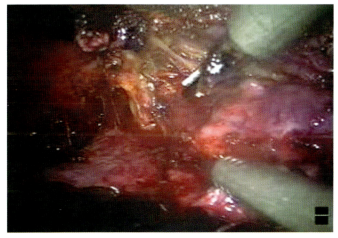

Figure 24-8. Dissection of the carina and hilum.

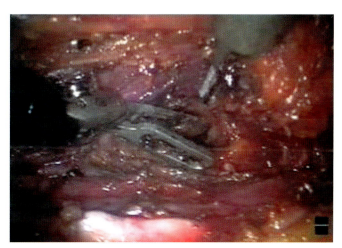

Figure 24-9. Dissection of the thoracic inlet.

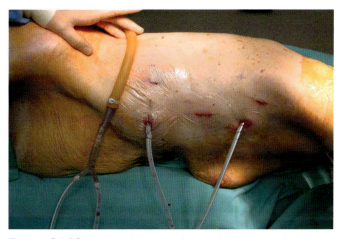

Figure 24-10. Drain placement during the thoracic phase.

Step 8. Isolation of the Cervical Esophagus

- Position the patient supinely, and reintubate with a single-lumen endotracheal tube. Turn the head upward and to the right, exposing the left side of the neck.
- Place the upper extremities by the sides, and keep the legs together.
- Make an oblique 5-cm transverse incision in the left neck 3 cm above the medial left clavicle.
- Continue the dissection deeply and medially toward the spine, transecting the omohyoid muscle for exposure.
- Encircle the previously mobilized and dissected esophagus with a Penrose drain, and pack the incision with an antibiotic-soaked surgical laparotomy pad to prevent carbon dioxide from later escaping from the peritoneal cavity.
- This initial dissection allows manipulation of the esophagus and unhindered withdrawal of the specimen later in the procedure.

Step 9. Abdominal-Phase Patient Positioning

- The patient is positioned supinely with the upper extremities placed by the sides and the legs kept together.

Step 10. Abdominal-Phase Port Placement

- A total of six abdominal puncture wounds are made. Place two 8-mm ports 8 cm subcostally at the right and left mid-clavicular lines for the robotic arms. Place an additional 12-mm trocar for the viewing port just cephalad to the umbilicus, maintaining a distance of 10 to 12 cm from either of the robotic arms (Figure 24-11).
- Place two additional 5-mm trocars beneath each costal margin in the anterior axillary line. Place another 12-mm port at the right mid-clavicular line at the umbilicus level (see Figure 24-11).

Step 11. Abdominal-Phase Docking

- Roll the robot into position. Place the robotic arms through the 8-mm trocars, and place the 30-degree down videoscope through the 12-mm viewing port.
- Inflate the abdomen with carbon dioxide to a pressure of 15 mm Hg.

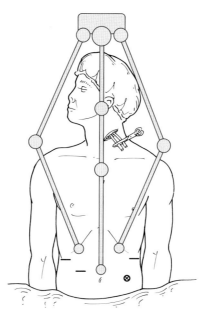

Figure 24-11. Port placement during the abdominal phase.

Step 12. Placement of a Feeding Jejunostomy

+ Before gastric dissection, place a laparoscopic feeding tube 20 cm from the ligament of Treitz, with transcutaneously placed 10-French T fasteners (Ross Flexiflow Lap J, Ross Products Division, Abbott Laboratories, Columbus, Ohio).

Step 13. Celiac Axis Lymphadenectomy

+ **Exposure:** Direct the camera toward the esophageal hiatus.
+ Set the videoscope in the 30-degree down position.
+ Lymph nodes are resected from the splenic hilum along the splenic artery to the origin of the left gastric artery and along the common hepatic artery up to the dissection plane completed in the thoracic phase of the procedure.

Step 14. Creation of a Gastric Conduit

+ **Exposure:** Direct the camera toward the esophageal hiatus.
+ Set the videoscope in the 30-degree down position.
+ Place a liver retractor exposing the esophageal hiatus through the right 5-mm accessory port.
+ Using the SonoSurg (Intuitive Surgical), transect the lesser omentum from the base of the liver up to the esophageal hiatus. Take the short gastric arteries, but preserve the right gastroepiploic arcade along its entirely to the right gastroepiploic vein at the transverse mesentery.
+ Transect the pyloric attachments to free the pylorus, allowing mobilization sufficient tissue to reach toward the esophageal hiatus. No Kocher maneuver or pyloroplasty is performed.
+ Approximately 4 to 5 cm cephalad from the origin of the right gastric artery along the lesser gastric curve, clear the gastric wall of perigastric tissue.
+ Using 8 to 10 firings of an Ethicon 45 × 4.1-mm linear endostapler, create a 4-cm-wide (from the greater curvature) right gastroepiploic arterial arcade–supplied gastric tube (Figure 24-12).
+ Suture the most cephalad aspect of the gastric tube to the most distal aspect of the specimen with two widely spaced figure-of-eight sutures (Figure 24-13).
+ Briefly discontinue the ventilator and chest drain suction, and use the Penrose drain encircling the esophagus at the neck as a handle to pull the specimen up through the neck incision.
+ Suture the intraperitoneal portion of the anterior gastric conduit serosa to each esophageal hiatus crus with two figure-of-eight, 3-0 Ethibond sutures to reduce the risk of later periconduit herniation.
+ Move the robot away form the patient to allow access to the left neck incision site. Close the abdominal trocar sites with 3-0 Vicryl sutures (Figure 24-14).

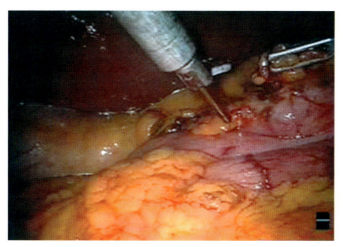

Figure 24-12. Gastric tube creation.

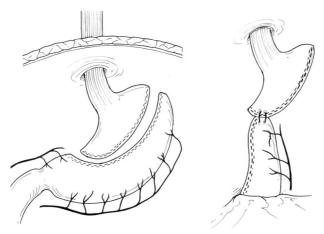

Figure 24-13. Attachment of the proximal gastric tube to the specimen.

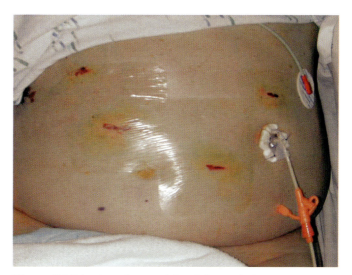

Figure 24-14. Completion of the abdominal phase.

Step 15. Esophagogastric Anastomosis
◆ At the incision in the left side of the neck, transect the specimen, and perform a stapled esophagogastrostomy. Create a side-to-side, functional end-to-end stapled anastomosis with a 45 × 4.1-mm linear endostapler and a 60 × 4.1-mm transverse stapler. This fashioned a 4 to 5 × 6-cm triangular anastomosis (Figure 24-15).
◆ Carefully place the nasogastric tube through the anastomosis before it is completed.
◆ Place a soft, multiholed drain in the neck beneath the platysma, avoiding the perimeter of the anastomosis.
◆ Close the cervical wound with interrupted 3-0 Vicryl sutures. A healed cervical wound is shown in Figure 24-16.

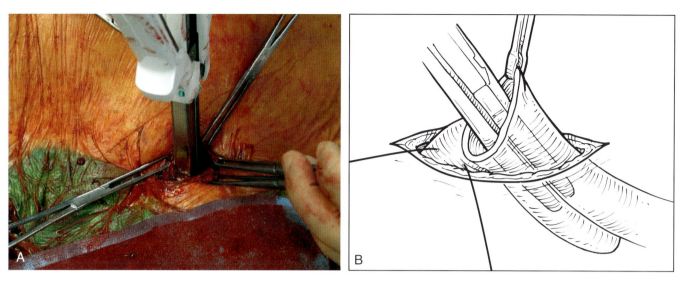

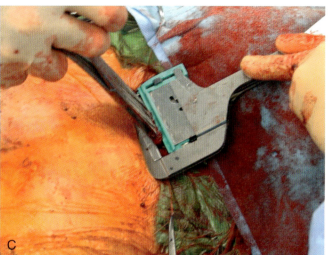

Figure 24-15. A-C, Neck anastomosis.

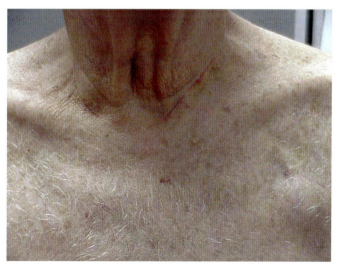

Figure 24-16. Healed cervical wound.

CHAPTER 25

VIDEO–ASSISTED THYMECTOMY—
VIDEO 25

Scott J. Swanson

Introduction

Thymectomy using a video-assisted thoracic surgical (VATS) approach is an excellent technique for patients with myasthenia gravis and small (<4 cm) thymomas that do not appear to invade other structures. It usually requires three right-sided ports, but if it is difficult to see the left phrenic nerve, a fourth left medial port may be needed.

Approach to Video-Assisted Thymectomy

Order of Operative Steps

The order of the steps of the operation is as follows: pericardial fat pad, pleura along phrenic nerve, right lower pole of thymus, open left pleura and left thymic pole, and left and right cervical poles.

Key Points

- Work from right to left and from inferior to superior.
- No manipulation of lung necessary.

 ## Video-Assisted Thymectomy (Video 25)

Step 1. Placement of Three Ports

- Position the patient supine with the arms over the head and an I-roll behind the patient (i.e., vertically behind the spine, horizontally behind the shoulders, and horizontally behind the hips) (Figure 25-1)
- Make the incisions.
  - ▲ Incision 1, made in the eighth intercostal space and along the mid-clavicular line, is for the camera.
  - ▲ Incision 2, made in the fourth intercostal space and medial to the breast (anterior clavicular line), is a working port.

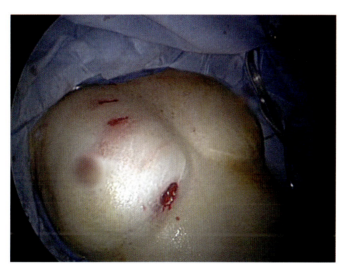

Figure 25-1. Incisions for a thymectomy performed as video-assisted thoracic surgery.

▲ Incision 3, made in the fifth intercostal space and medial to the breast (anterior clavicular line), is a working port.
▲ Incision 4 (optional) is made in the left seventh intercostal space and anterior to the clavicular line.

Step 2. Initial Dissection

◆ **Exposure:** Gravity makes the lung fall posteriorly, out of the way.
◆ Aim the thoracoscope superiorly, and point the lens toward the mediastinum.
◆ A grasper through incision 3 lifts the pleura anterior to the phrenic nerve. The Harmonic scalpel opens the mediastinal pleura parallel to the right phrenic nerve pedicle and approximately 2 mm anterior to it (Figure 25-2A).
◆ Carry this dissection superiorly to the origin of the superior vena cava, where the left innominate vein and right innominate vein join (Figure 25-2B).

Step 3. Dissection of the Right Lower Pole of the Thymus

◆ **Exposure:** Gravity makes the lung fall posteriorly, out of the way.
◆ Aim the thoracoscope superiorly, and point the lens toward the mediastinum.
◆ A ring forceps through incision 2 holds the thymus as the Endokittner (Ethicon Endosurgery, Cincinnati, Ohio) bluntly sweeps the right pole of the thymus from the pericardium (Figure 25-3A).
◆ If vascular adhesions are encountered, use the Harmonic scalpel (Ethicon Endosurgery) to control them (Figure 25-3B).
◆ Take diaphragmatic fat with the inferior aspect of the right thymic pole by dividing attachments to the diaphragm with the Harmonic scalpel or by sweeping them off bluntly with the Ethicon Endokittner.
◆ Carry this dissection to the midline (i.e., level of sternum) (Figure 25-3C).

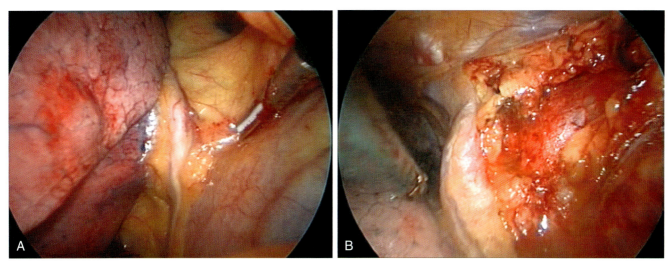

Figure 25-2. **A,** The Harmonic scalpel starts the dissection anterior to the phrenic nerve. **B,** The thymus is dissected off the surface of the pericardium.

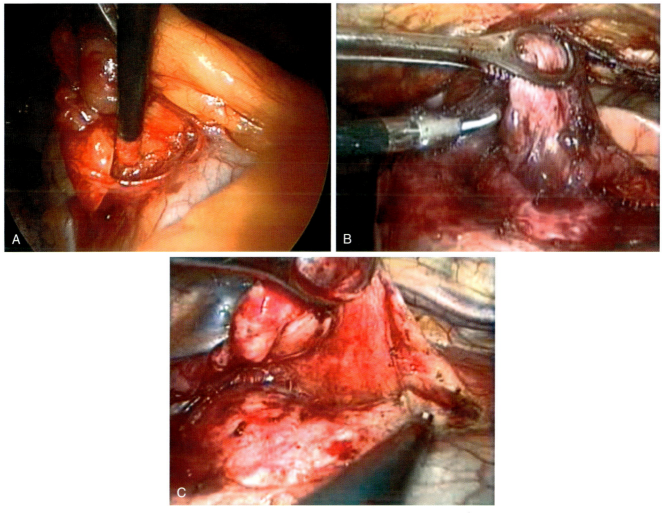

Figure 25-3. **A,** Endokittner bluntly dissects the thymus away from the pericardium. **B,** The Harmonic scalpel transects small vessels. **C,** Blunt dissection of the thymus off the surface of the pericardium.

Step 4. Dissection of the Left Lower Pole of the Thymus
- **Exposure:** Gravity makes the lung fall posteriorly, out of the way.
- Aim the thoracoscope superiorly, and point the lens toward the mediastinum.
- At level of sternum, bluntly create the plane between peristernal tissue (including the mammary pedicle) and the left-sided mediastinal pleura.
- When mediastinal pleura is clearly identified over the left lung, open the pleura with the Harmonic scalpel (Figure 25-4A and B).
- After the left thymic pole is clearly identified, begin dissection along medial left diaphragmatic surface, including the diaphragmatic fat, to ensure that the entire thymus is resected.
- Use Harmonic scalpel to open the mediastinal pleura 2 mm anterior to the left phrenic pedicle (i.e., similar to dissection on right side) (Figure 25-4C).
- Carry the dissection up to the level of the left innominate vein (Figure 25-4D).
- If there is any issue regarding visualization of the left phrenic pedicle add 4th port in left 7th intercostal space in anterior clavicular line. Put camera in this port and ask anesthesiologists to intermittently hold ventilation to visualize structures (this is necessary <20% of the time) (Figure 25-4E).

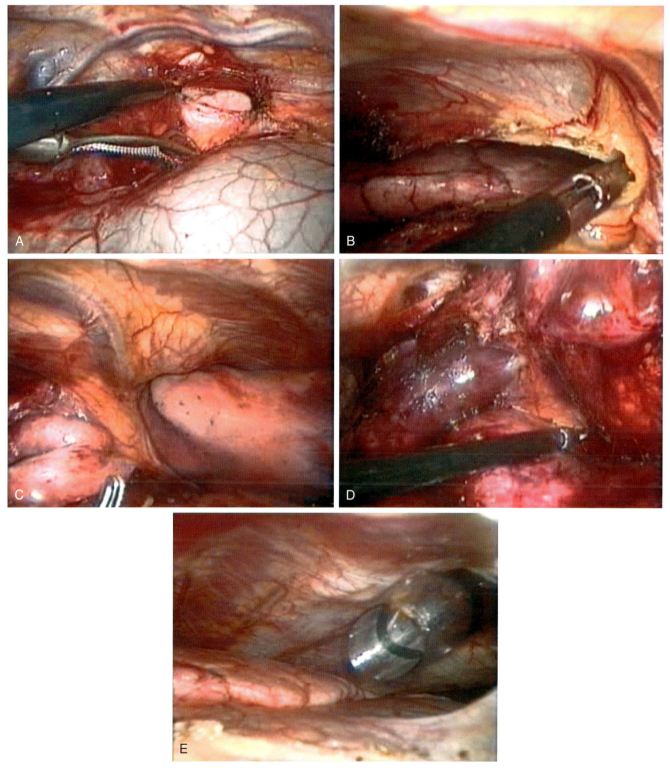

Figure 25-4. A, Opening the contralateral pleura. **B,** The Harmonic scalpel resects the left pericardial fat pad. **C,** The Harmonic scalpel dissects just anteriorly to the left phrenic nerve. **D,** Dissection proceeds along the surface of the innominate vein. **E,** Placement of a trocar into the left pleural space facilitates visualization of the left phrenic nerve.

Step 5. Identification of the Cervical Thymic Poles Superficial and Superior to the Left Innominate Vein

- **Exposure:** Gravity makes the lung fall posteriorly, out of the way.
- Aim the thoracoscope medially, and point the lens superiorly.
- Open the fascial layer over the left and right cervical thymic poles, and begin blunt dissection with the Endokittner (Figure 25-5A).
- Divide any draining vessels with the Harmonic scalpel.
- When the poles have been brought down to the level of the innominate vein, identify the draining veins of the body of the thymus into the innominate, and divide these veins with the Harmonic scalpel, or clip and cut them (depending on the surgeon's preference) (Figure 25-5B and C).
- Occasionally, the right internal mammary vein at the juncture with the innominate vein prevents visualization of the cervical thymic poles. It can be clipped and divided to open up the space into the neck.
- After the vascular supply to the cervical poles has been controlled, each pole can be teased out of the neck (Figure 25-5D and E).

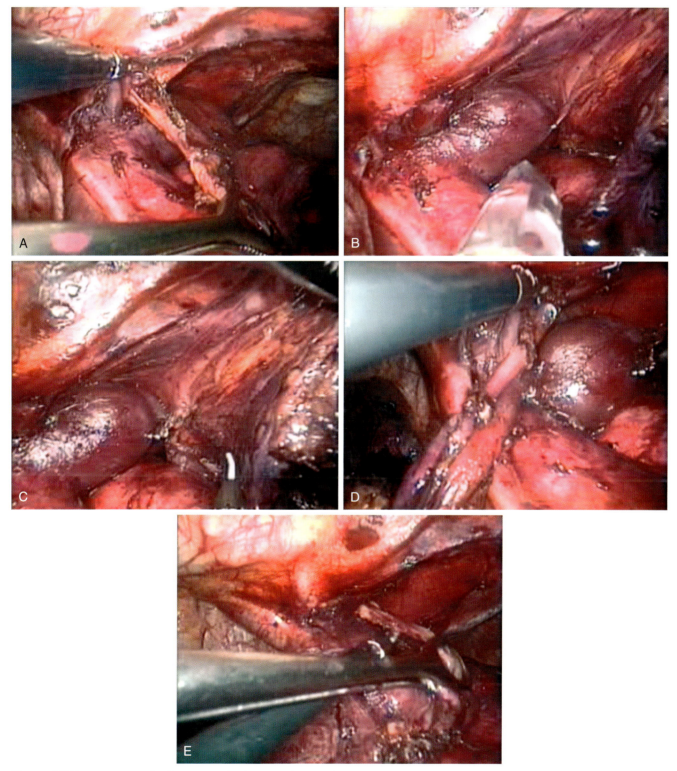

Figure 25-5. A, Opening the fascia over the thymic poles. **B**, The thymic veins are divided between clips using scissors. **C**, Thymic veins have been clipped. **D**, Mobilization of the right thymic pole from the neck. **E**, Mobilization of the left thymic pole from the neck.

Step 6. Thymus Retrieval

- **Exposure:** Gravity makes the lung fall posteriorly, out of the way.
- Aim the thoracoscope inferiorly, and point the lens toward the mediastinum.
- At this point, the entire thymus should be freed, along with the surrounding mediastinal and diaphragmatic fat. Place the specimen in a retrieval bag, and remove it from the chest through incision 2 (Figure 25-6).

Step 7. Chest Tube

- **Exposure:** Gravity makes the lung fall posteriorly, out of the way.
- Aim the thoracoscope inferiorly, and point the lens toward the mediastinum.
- Inspect the thymic bed for hemostasis and completeness of dissection (Figure 25-7A).
- Place a 19-French Blake drain into the chest through the camera port, and drape in a large C shape so that the pleural spaces and mediastinum are well drained (Figure 25-7B).

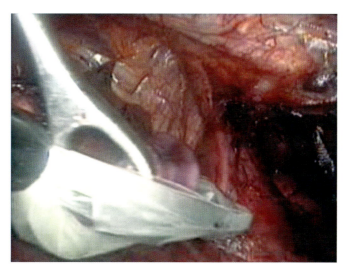

Figure 25-6. The thymus is removed and placed in a bag.

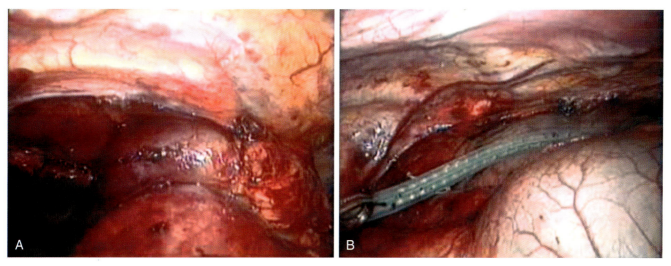

Figure 25-7. A, Empty anterior mediastinum. **B,** Chest tube drainage of the mediastinum.

Miscellaneous Topics

CHAPTER 26

LUNG VOLUME REDUCTION SURGERY — VIDEO 26

Robert J. McKenna, Jr.

Introduction

Compared with maximal medical management, lung volume reduction surgery (LVRS) has improved quality of life, pulmonary function, exercise tolerance, and survival for selected patients.[1] Although LVRS can be performed as video-assisted thoracic surgery (VATS) or a median sternotomy with the same morbidity, mortality, and benefits, the VATS approach costs less and provides earlier recovery.[2]

Patients who are candidates for LVRS are symptomatic despite maximal medical management, including inhalers, oxygen supplementation, and pulmonary rehabilitation. The latter helps to screen and treat patients. Patients with severe emphysema are deconditioned, and rehabilitation reconditions the leg muscles and reduces dyspnea. Better-conditioned patients are better prepared to cooperate with their postoperative tasks, such as immediate ambulation and use of the incentive spirometer, to reduce respiratory complications. Patients who do not cooperate well or fail at rehabilitation are poor candidates for LVRS. The most important selection factor is a heterogeneous pattern of emphysema identified on computed tomography (CT) and lung perfusion scanning.

Approach to Video-Assisted Lung Volume Reduction Surgery

Order of Operative Steps

Video-assisted LVRS is performed most commonly as a staged, bilateral procedure with the patient in the lateral decubitus position. Unless there is a massive air leak after the first side is completed, the patient is turned over for LVRS on the opposite side. The area to be resected is determined by the preoperative workup. The preoperative CT and perfusion scans to determine the area to be resected (usually the upper lobes). These areas do not deflate well intraoperatively because of poor elastic recoil.

Key Points

- Work anteriorly to posteriorly over the top of the lung.
- Resection starts in the anterior segment of the upper lobe, just above the middle lobe on the right and the lingula on the left.
- Tiny air leaks may take weeks to heal. Limit the manipulation and contact with the lung. A severely emphysematous lung is very soft, and minimal contact with the lung, such as touching it with a stapler, can make a hole in the lung.
- Repeat operations to close an air leak are rarely indicated.

Video-Assisted Lung Volume Reduction Surgery (Video 26)

Step 1. Incisions

- Incision 1: Through the sixth intercostal space in the mid-clavicular line, make a 2-cm incision as far inferiorly and medially as possible. This is usually one space below the inframammary crease. The dissection through this incision is angled posteriorly through the chest wall (away from the pericardium) so that instruments through this incision are automatically directed posteriorly toward the major fissure, not toward the heart. Check for adhesions with a finger through the incision (Figure 26-1).
- Incision 2: Through the ninth intercostal space in the mid-clavicular line, make a 5-mm incision for the 5-mm trocar and a 30-degree thoracoscope.
- Incision 3: Make a 2-cm incision in the fourth intercostal space in the mid-axillary line.

Step 2. Decompression of Apical Bullous Disease

- **Exposure:** Retract the right upper lobe apically.
- Aim the thoracoscope anteriorly with the 30-degree lens pointed superiorly.
- The bullous disease of the apex of the lung does not decompress well. With the Metzenbaum scissors (or electrocautery) through incision 3, cut into the parenchyma of the right upper lobe to decompress the bullous parenchyma of the upper lobe (Figure 26-2).

Step 3. Lung Resection

- **Exposure:** Retract the right lower lobe directly apically.
- Aim the thoracoscope anteriorly with the 30-degree lens pointed apically.
- As with any operation, exposure is the key (Figures 26-3 and 26-4). With a ring forceps through incision 3, hold the lung to line up the parenchyma for the stapler that passes through incision 1.
- The buttress on the stapler reduces the air leaks when the lung is stapled. Do not manipulate the stapler much, because this may tear the lung and cause air leaks. Before introducing the stapler, align the lung so that the stapler slides easily across the lung.
- If the lung is aligned incorrectly, the stapler will be oblique to the lung and can create a hole in the lung.

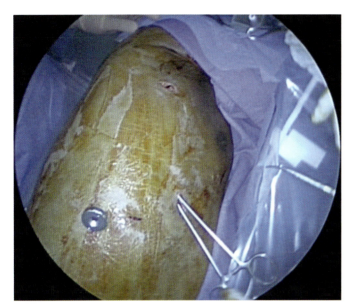

Figure 26-1. Incisions for lung volume reduction surgery.

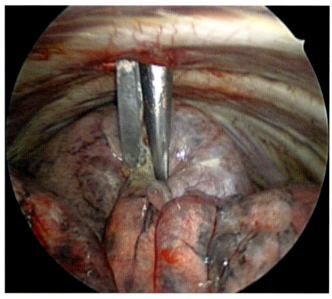

Figure 26-2. Metzenbaum scissors cutting the parenchyma of the upper lobe to decompress the upper lobe for resection.

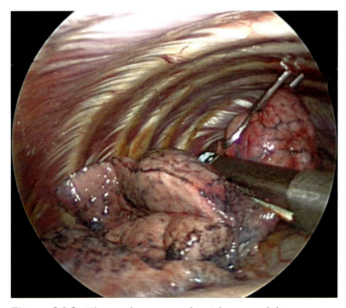

Figure 26-3. The stapler crosses the right upper lobe to start the lung volume reduction surgery.

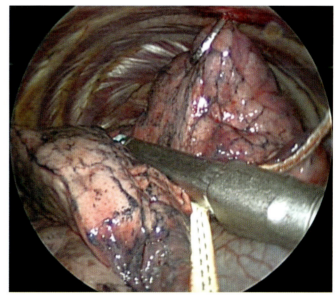

Figure 26-4. The stapler continues the lung volume reduction surgery across the right upper lobe.

Step 4. Completion of Surgery

- **Exposure:** Retract the right lower lobe directly apically.
- Aim the thoracoscope anteriorly with the 30-degree lens pointed apically.
- The buttressed stapler continues across the lung approximately 3 to 4 cm from the minor and major fissures laterally and close to the hilum medially. As the stapler is fired, move the ring forceps holding the lung closer to the area of lung that has just been stapled (Figures 26-5 to 26-7).
- When stapling is completed, cut the bridge of the buttress material that holds the specimen to the lung that remains (Figure 26-8).

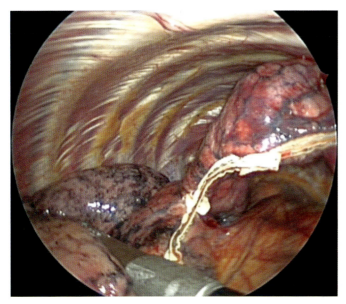

Figure 26-5. Proximity of the staple line to the hilum.

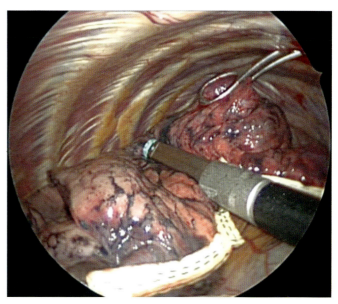

Figure 26-6. The staple line continues parallel to and approximately 3 to 4 cm from the fissure.

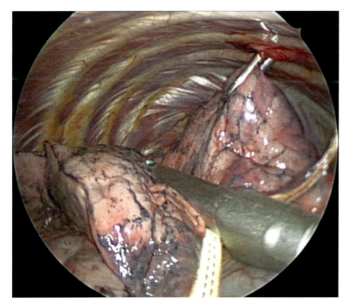

Figure 26-7. Final firing of the stapler across the lung for lung volume reduction surgery.

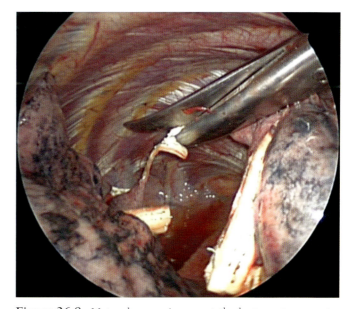

Figure 26-8. Metzenbaum scissors cut the buttress to separate the lung to be removed.

Step 5. Specimen Removal

- **Exposure:** The lung does not need to be retracted because the LVRS has removed enough tissue to provide excellent exposure of the pleural cavity.
- Aim the thoracoscope anteriorly with the 30-degree lens pointed apically.
- Pull the lung specimen through incision 1 with a ring forceps (Figure 26-9).

Postoperative Care

- Extubate the patient in the operating room.
- Pain relief is imperative to allow patients to ambulate, cough, and use the incentive spirometer. Use an epidural catheter initially and then narcotics for pain relief. Use a patient-controlled analgesia (PCA) pump if the epidural is not working well. Pain must be controlled immediately after the operation so that uncontrolled pain does not lead to pneumonia.
- Respiratory care is essential.
  - ▲ Early ambulation twice daily in the hallway reduces the risk of pulmonary complications.
  - ▲ Aggressively use nebulizer treatments with chest physiotherapy.
  - ▲ No suction is applied to the chest tubes.
  - ▲ When the chest tube drainage is low, attach Heimlich valves to the chest tubes if there is still an air leak. This facilitates ambulation.
  - ▲ Even if patients do not retain carbon dioxide before the operation, they often have carbon dioxide pressures in the mid-60s (mm Hg) after LVRS.
- Arrhythmias, especially atrial fibrillation, occur in about 20% of patients. The cause often is hypoxemia and atelectasis.
- Gastrointestinal complications are common. If the patient has not had a bowel movement by day 2, aggressively use laxatives. Air swallowing, pain medicine, and the epidural can cause severe abdominal distention and even colonic perforation.

References

1. Naunheim K, et al and the NETT Research Group. Long-Term Follow-up of Patients Receiving Lung-Volume-Reduction Surgery Versus Medical Therapy for Servere Emphysema. Ann Thorac Surg; 82: 431–443, 2006.
2. McKenna Rj, et al for the National Emphysema Treatment Trial (NETT) Research Group. National Emphysema Treatment Trial: A Comparision of Median Sternotomy versus VATS for Lung Volume Reduction Surgery. J Thorac Cardiovasc Surg 2004: 127; 1350–1360.

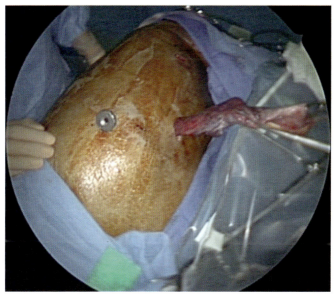

Figure 26-9. The lung volume reduction surgery specimen is removed through incision 1.

CHAPTER 27

RESECTION OF PULMONARY BLEBS AND BULLAE—VIDEO 27

Cynthia S. Chin and Scott J. Swanson

Introduction

One of the earliest and most widespread uses for video-assisted thoracic surgery (VATS) was for treatment of patients with spontaneous pneumothoraces. Bleb resection by VATS has become a standard procedure, but the method for pleurodesis remains controversial. Studies of treatment of spontaneous pneumothorax have not been able to show one method of pleurodesis to be more successful than another. Video-assisted resection of bullae is part of lung volume reduction surgery for the treatment end-stage emphysema. Indications for this type of operation are too extensive to discuss in this chapter, which reviews important points for bleb and bullae resection.

Approach to Video-Assisted Resection of Pulmonary Blebs and Bullae

Order of Operative Steps

The order of the steps of the operation is lysis of adhesions, visualization and palpation of the bleb, resection planning, resection with pericardial strips, and checking for air leaks. The final step of pleurodesis is discussed in Chapter 21.

Key Points
- Adhesions may be present secondary to previous pneumothoraces and pleural irritation.
- Lung malignancy has been found within blebs and bullae.

 ## Video-Assisted Resection of Pulmonary Blebs and Bullae (Video 27)

Step 1. Port Placement
- Place the camera port in the seventh intercostal space in the anterior axillary line; it is modified depending on heart size.
- Place the access port in the fourth intercostal space in the mid-axillary line.
- Place the posterior port in the sixth intercostal space just inferior to the tip of the scapula.

Step 2. Lysis of Adhesions

◆ **Exposure:** Retract the lung away from the adhesion.
◆ Aim the thoracoscope anteriorly with the 30-degree lens pointed toward the adhesion.
◆ Patients may have pleural adhesions from the pleural irritation that occurs with a previous pneumothorax. Lyse these adhesions so the entire lung can be mobilized (Figure 27-1).
◆ Adhesions to the lateral and posterior walls are evident with lung isolation. However, adhesions on the medial wall may be less obvious.
◆ If there is tension on the lung as it is mobilized, be wary of medial adhesions. Take down these adhesions with an electrocautery or ultrasonic dissector.
◆ Failure to recognize an adhesion may lead to torn visceral pleura. In this patient population, this may become the source of a prolonged postoperative air leak.

Step 3. Visualization and Palpation of Blebs

◆ **Exposure:** Place ring forceps through the posterior port to mobilize the lung. Palpate the lung parenchyma with a finger through the anterior incision.
◆ Aim the thoracoscope anteriorly with the 30-degree lens pointed posteriorly.
◆ After the lung is free of adhesions, palpate it for parenchymal lesions. Lung cancers are associated with emphysematous bullae.
◆ Because the anterior rib space usually is larger, palpation is best achieved by mobilizing the lung toward the anterior port with a ring forceps placed through the posterior port.
◆ Palpate the lung with a finger through the anterior port (Figure 27-2).
◆ For better mobilization, it may help to divide the inferior pulmonary ligament at this time.

Step 4. Resection Planning

◆ **Exposure:** Retract the lung with a ring forceps through the posterior port. Place a second pair of ring forceps through the anterior port to plan the line of resection.
◆ Aim the thoracoscope anteriorly with the 30-degree lens pointed posteriorly.
◆ The two ring forceps are used in the anterior and posterior ports to help plan the resection.
◆ One ring should hold the lung, and the other ring should be placed where the stapler will be fired.
◆ Adjustments can be made more easily with a ring forceps than with the larger stapler.
◆ Compress the lung with a ring forceps to allow the stapler to slide across the lung more readily.

Step 5. Resection with Pericardial Strips

◆ **Exposure:** A ring forceps through the posterior port stabilizes the lung.
◆ Aim the thoracoscope anteriorly with the 30-degree lens pointed posteriorly.
◆ It is best to bring the stapler through the anterior access port because the rib spaces are wider anteriorly and because there is less chance of postoperative neuralgia from the relatively large and rigid stapler.
◆ Reinforce the staple lines with bovine pericardium or polytetrafluorethylene if the lung parenchyma is very emphysematous (Figure 27-3). In certain patient populations, the use of these materials has been shown to decrease postoperative air leaks and chest tube duration.

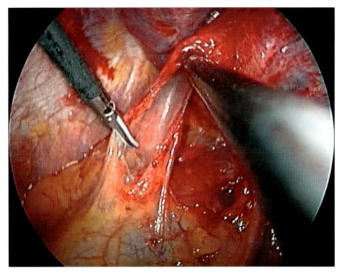

Figure 27-1. Lysis of adhesions with an ultrasonic scalpel.

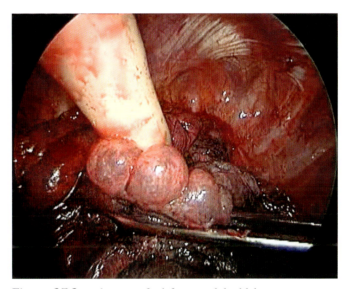

Figure 27-2. Palpation of a left upper lobe bleb.

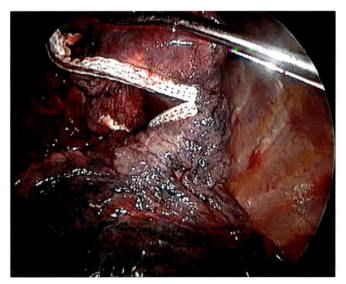

Figure 27-3. Wedge resection of a bleb using pericardial strips.

- For patients with a spontaneous pneumothorax caused by an isolated bleb, we usually do not reinforce the staple line unless the lung parenchyma appears to be abnormal. For patients who have more diffuse lung disease, we buttress the staple line.
- After the bleb is resected, bring it out through the anterior access port in an EndoCATCH bag (Covidien, Mansfield, Mass), to protect the port site in case of an incidental lung cancer or subclinical infection, such as *Mycobacteria avium-intracellulare.*

Step 6. Checking for Air Leaks

- **Exposure:** Bring a dental pledget on a long Allis clamp through the posterior port to gently hold the staple line in water while the lung is reinflated.
- Aim the thoracoscope anteriorly with the 30-degree lens pointed posteriorly.
- To check for residual air leaks, place a dental pledget on a long Allis clamp, and bring it in through the posterior port. Use this to hold the area of interest down when the lung is reinflated.
- Instill water in the chest cavity and reinflate the lung.
- If there is no air leak, isolate the lung again, and place two chest tubes.
- Place the camera in the posterior port to confirm good reinflation of the lung.

CHAPTER 28

THORACOSCOPIC SYMPATHECTOMY

Mark J. Krasna

Introduction

Thoracoscopic sympathectomy has been used for the treatment of sympathetic dysfunction since it was first described by Kux and colleagues in the 1940s.[1] With the advent of video-assisted thoracic surgery (VATS), the procedure has become more widely applied.[2] VATS allows excellent visual acuity and the possibility of doing the procedure more quickly and with fewer complications. It is the most effective treatment for palmar hyperhidrosis.

Thoracic sympathectomy is indicated for a variety of sympathetic disorders, but it is most commonly performed for hyperhidrosis. Reflex sympathetic dystrophy, upper extremity ischemia, Raynaud's disease, debilitating facial blushing, and splanchnicectomy for pancreatic pain are less common indications.

Patients undergoing thoracoscopic sympathectomy usually have tried nonoperative therapy, such as topical agents (e.g., Drysol [aluminum hydroxide]) or iontophoresis (if the patient can tolerate the side effects of tingling and electrical shocks). Unfortunately, the effects usually wear off, and patients often cannot tolerate the uncomfortable sensation. Antidepressants or other psychotropic medications have not provided significant benefit. Beta-blockers and cholinergics may provide short-term improvement, but most patients stop these medications because of the side effects, including fatigue, dry mouth, and bradycardia.

Nomenclature

Many terms have been used in different studies to describe the procedure that is performed. Unfortunately, the terminology used in international papers is inconsistent and often leads to confusion. The following glossary has been proposed and corresponds to the diagrams and intraoperative photographs found in the chapter.

- Ablation: procedures in which the chain is destroyed using electrocautery or laser without directed division.
- Clipping: placing one clip above the ganglion; placing one clip each above and below the ganglion; placing a clip across the nerve over the middle of the rib; or placing clips above or below the ganglion.[3]
- Sympathectomy: procedure in which the sympathetic chain is resected, ablated, or divided.
- Sympathicotomy: division of the sympathetic chain without removal of any section thereof. Unless otherwise specified, this excludes ablation techniques that are done without a directed division of the chain.

- R2 sympathectomy or sympathicotomy: division or resection of the chain overlying the second (R2 rib) and third rib (R3). This division accomplishes isolation of the R2 ganglion, which is found in between the two cuts (Figure 28-1). This nomenclature should be used for all subsequent levels; for example, R3 sympathectomy or sympathicotomy means division of the nerve chain over the third and fourth ribs, achieving R3 ganglion isolation.
- Thoracoscopic procedure: done with any means of thoracoscopy, including video-assisted and standard eyepiece-assisted procedures.
- Video-assisted thoracoscopic surgery (VATS): procedure using a video camera to help with visualization of the intrathoracic cavity.

Approach to Video-Assisted Thoracoscopic Sympathectomy

Choice of Transection Level

The transection level is based on the recommendations of the Society of Thoracic Surgeons Workforce on Hyperhidrosis. Choice of the appropriate level depends on the location of the primary symptoms:
- Facial sweating: The R2 level is isolated by dividing over the R2 and R3 ribs. Alternatively, some surgeons treat facial sweating or blushing with division of the chain over the R2 rib, taking care to avoid injuring the stellate ganglion, although the lower third of the stellate ganglion can be transected without causing Horner's syndrome.
- Palmar sweating: Transect the chain at R3 and R4.
- Axillary sweating: Transect the chain at R4 and R5.
- Reflex sympathetic dystrophy or thoracic outlet syndrome: A R2 to R3 sympathectomy is performed.
- Chronic pancreatic pain: Sympathectomy and splanchnicectomy are performed from R4 to R10 levels.

Key Points

- Avoid damage to the underlying periosteum, because it can cause severe discomfort and sunburn-like pain in the postoperative period.
- Avoid the sympathetic chain above the level of the R2 ganglion to prevent Horner's syndrome. Avoid cauterizing the cut proximal end of the R2 ganglion.

Video-Assisted Thoracoscopic Sympathectomy

Step 1. Setup for Sympathectomy

- Use general anesthesia with a single-lumen endotracheal tube and carbon dioxide insufflation to decompress the lung.
- Place the patient in a supine position with arms extended or in a semi-Fowler position.
- The arms are placed on armboards and rotated out (adducted) but left in a neutral position with padding under the ulnar nerve at the elbow to avoid postoperative neuralgia.
- Place a roll under the spine so the skin preparation can be done from the right posterior axillary line to the left posterior axillary line.
- Use a single 1-cm incision in the second intercostal space in the anterior axillary line, just posterior to the pectoralis muscle if the procedure is performed with a 0-degree, 10-mm thoracoscope, or use two 3-mm trocars in the second and fourth intercostal spaces in the anterior axillary line.

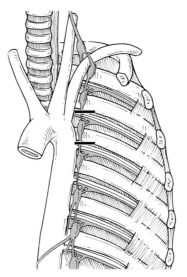

Figure 28-1. The sympathetic chain is transected above and below the third ganglion to correct palmar hyperhidrosis.

Step 2. Exposure of the Sympathetic Chain

- Stop the ventilation, and detach the ventilator from the endotracheal tube.
- Pass a Veress needle through the inferior incision. Carbon dioxide is insufflated at a rate of 2 L/min with a pressure limit of 10 mm Hg.[4]
- After 400 mL of carbon dioxide has been insufflated, insert the second trocar to confirm that the lung is deflating.
- When the lung has deflated sufficiently for exposure of the desired level of the sympathetic chain, resume ventilation.

Step 3. Sympathectomy

- **Exposure:** The apex of the chest is exposed as the insufflation deflates the lung.
- Aim the thoracoscope anteriorly with the 30-degree lens pointed apically.
- Pass the hook electrocautery probes (2, 3, or 5 mm) through the working thoracoscope or the superior trocar.
- Identify the sympathetic chain over the middle of the rib where the rib head articulates with the transverse processes. Incise the parietal pleura first, and separate the lateral edges of the chain.
- With electrocautery, cut the chain, and coagulate the divided ends of the chain.
- Complete division of the sympathetic chain, including the nerve of Kuntz (identified in about 20% of cases), must be achieved to avoid a recurrence.
- For the clip procedure, encircle the chain with an L-shaped hook electrocautery, and mobilize the chain for about 1 cm.

Step 4. Lung Reexpansion

- The thoracoscope is pointed apically.
- Insufflation is stopped.
- After ensuring proper hemostasis, place a small catheter (chest tube or 12- to 20 French red rubber catheter) in the chest through the trocar. Reinflate the lung, and allow exsufflation of air and carbon dioxide from the chest.
- Alternatively, open the trocars to allow egress of the air from the chest and to allow the lung to expand as the anesthesiologist reexpands the lung. Place the thoracoscope back in the trocar to ensure that the lung is fully expanded. A large breath is held as the trocars are removed.
- Close the incisions with a subcutaneous 3-0 absorbable and 4-0 subcuticular suture.
- If 2- or 3-mm trocars are used, Johnson & Johnson's Dermabond (Ethicon, Cincinnati, OH) may be used to seal the skin without sutures.
- The same procedure is then performed on the opposite side.

Results

In a series of 396 consecutive procedures (synchronous bilateral in 388 patients, right side alone in 6, left side alone in 1, staged in 1) included 191 (48%) men and 206 (52%) women. The mean age was 29 years (range, 9 to 65 years). Median hospital stay was 0.5 day (range, 0.5 to 3 days). Median follow-up was 2.6 years (range, 2 months to 9 years). The indications were hyperhidrosis in 370 patients, facial blushing in 21, Raynaud's in 3, digital ischemia in 2, and reflex sympathetic dystrophy in 1 patient. Compensatory sweating occurred in 40% ($n = 81$ of 202).[5]

A series of 453 patients showed excellent (74.2%) or good (19.6%) quality of life at 5 years of follow-up.[6] In another series of 222 patients, excellent results were reported for more than 90% and compensatory sweating for 85% of patients.[7] Results of these two studies suggested that division of the R2 ganglion should be avoided because compensatory sweating developed in 48% of patients when R2 was transected but in only

16% when R2 was not transected. When severe compensatory sweating developed, more than 50% of patients wished that they had not undergone the procedure.

Miller and Force[8] described a novel approach to thoracoscopic sympathectomy. They devised a method to screen patients who would be more likely to develop compensatory sweating. They injected the nerve at the planned operative level and reassessed patients after they emerged from anesthesia.[8] If the patients benefitted from the injection and did not develop intolerable compensatory sweating, they subsequently underwent sympathectomy.

Tools have been devised to evaluate quality of life (QOL) in terms of objective response, satisfaction, and complications after thoracoscopic sympathectomy. In 1998, Krasna and colleagues proposed a 4-point scoring system of the severity and social impact after thoracoscopic sympathectomy.[9] Kwong described a QOL index,[10] and Ribas and associates used a standard short-form health survey (SF-36).[11] Each of these systems attempts to quantitate the positive and negative results of this procedure for making decisions and assessing costs.

Complications and Repeat Operations

Common side effects include paresthesias (1%), pneumothorax (1%), bleeding, infection (1%), and incisional pain similar to post-thoracotomy pain (3%). Uncommon complications include chylothorax and esophageal and lung injury. Rare cases of severe bradycardia, Horner's syndrome, and severe compensatory sweating have occurred.

Because compensatory sweating, which occurs in 20% to 80% of cases, is the most common side effect, it should be explained to the patient as an expected outcome of this operation. Of these patients, 2% to 20% have severe, disabling compensatory sweating that results in enough dissatisfaction that they regret having the operation.

An unusual complication that should be discussed with the patient preoperatively is Horner's syndrome, which occurs in less than 5% of patients. Decreased baseline heart rate and a decrease in the response to stress are expected to some degree in all patients.[12] This is a possible cause of postoperative dysfunction and should be cautiously investigated. All of these complications should be discussed with the patient before surgery.

Reoperation after prior thoracic procedures is not contraindicated, as reported by Kim and colleagues.[13] In this series, even patients with previous open and thoracoscopic surgery did not have adhesions that prevented successful thoracoscopic sympathectomy.

References

1. Kux M: Thoracic endoscopic sympathectomy in palmar and axillary hyperhidrosis, *Arch Surg* 113:264–266, 1978.
2. Göthberg C, Drott, Claes G: Thoracoscopic sympathicotomy for hyperhidrosis–surgical technique, complications and side effects, *Eur J Surg Suppl* 572:51–53, 1994.
3. Lin TS, Huang LC, Wang NP, Chang CC: Video-assisted thoracoscopic T2 sympathetic block by clipping for palmar hyperhidrosis: analysis of 52 cases, *J Laparoendosc Adv Surg Tech A* 11:59–62, 2001.
4. Wolfer RS, Krasna MJ, Hasnain JU, McLaughlin JS: Hemodynamic effects of carbon dioxide insufflation during thoracoscopy, *Ann Thorac Surg* 58:404–408, 1994.
5. Kwong K, Krasna M: Clinical experience in 397 consecutive thoracoscopic sympathectomies, *Ann Thorac Surg* 80:1063–1066, 2005.
6. Milanez de Campos J, Kauffman P, et al: Quality of life, before and after thoracic sympathectomy: report on 378 operated patients, *Ann Thorac Surg* 76:886–891, 2003.
7. Dewey TM, Herbert MA, Hill SL, et al: One-year follow-up after thoracoscopic sympathectomy for hyperhidrosis: outcomes and consequences, *Ann Thorac Surg* 81:1227–1232, 2006.
8. Miller DL, Force SD: Temporary thoracoscopic sympathetic block for hyperhidrosis, *Ann Thorac Surg* 85:1211–1214, 2008.
9. Krasna M, Demmy T, McKenna R, Mack M: Thoracoscopic sympathectomy: the U.S. experience, *Eur J Surg Suppl* 580:19–21, 1998.
10. Krasna MJ, Jiao X, Sonett J, et al: Thoracoscopic sympathectomy, *Surg Laparosc Endosc Percutan Tech* 10:314–318, 2000.
11. Ribas Milanez de Campos J, Kauffman P, Wolosker N, et al: Axillary hyperhidrosis: T3/T4 versus T4 thoracic sympathectomy in a series of 276 cases, *J Laparoendosc Adv Tech A* 16:598–603, 2006.
12. Drott C, Claes G, Paszkowski P: Cardiac effects of endoscopic electrocautery of the upper sympathetic chain, *Eur J Surg* 572 (Suppl):65–70, 1994.
13. Kim DH, Paik HC, Lee DY: Video assisted thoracoscopic re-sympathetic surgery in the treatment of re-sweating hyperhidrosis, *Eur J Cardiothorac Surg* 27:741–744, 2005.

CHAPTER 29

FIRST RIB RESECTION FOR THORACIC OUTLET SYNDROME — VIDEO 29-1

Randall Kevin Wolf and Robert J. McKenna, Jr.

Introduction

There are several surgical approaches for thoracic outlet syndrome (TOS). The video-assisted thoracic surgical (VATS) approach has several advantages. The shoulder does not have to be lifted and held for an extended time, the exposure is very good, and cutaneous nerves in the axilla are not disturbed.

Treatment of TOS requires resection of the first rib. TOS refers to compression of the subclavian vessels or the brachial plexus, or both, by the first rib and adjacent structures at the superior aperture of the chest.[1] Sir James Paget in 1875 in London and von Schroetter in 1884 in Vienna reported thrombosis of the subclavian vein caused by TOS. This vascular form of TOS is known as Paget–von Schroetter syndrome. However, the most common symptoms are neurologic and are related to compression of the brachial plexus in the distribution of the ulnar nerve.

Approach to Video-Assisted First Rib Resection

Order of Operative Steps

The order of the steps for video-assisted first rib resection is as follows: lateral decubitus position with the arm elevated on an airplane support, complete mobilization of the rib, excision of a 1-cm piece of the rib in the mid-clavicular line, and removal of the anterior and posterior pieces of the rib.[3]

Key Points

- Count and visualize the ribs carefully. On thoracoscopic examination, the first rib can be easily identified in the "roof" of the thorax. It can be palpated indirectly using an endokittner and can be clearly visualized.
- On the left, the subclavian artery is easily visualized on the thoracoscopic examination.
- Mobilize the entire rib before opening the pleura, because the carbon dioxide decompression of the lung is lost after opening the pleura, and the operative field is ecchymotic after the pleura is opened.

- When the rib has been mobilized as much as possible, excise a 1-cm piece of the rib in the mid-axillary line. This allows caudal displacement of the rib to complete the mobilization to the sternum anteriorly and to the vertebral bodies posteriorly.
- The ribs can be disarticulated or cut, but cutting seems to cause less pain.
- Care must be taken in developing the plane of dissection, and dissecting anterior to the vein initially is recommended.
- Care should be taken to observe and preserve the internal mammary artery anteriorly and the sympathetic chain posteriorly to the borders of the first rib.
- Port sites are best placed at some distance from the target to allow adequate manipulation of the instruments in a comfortable arc.

Video-Assisted First Rib Resection (Video 29-1)

Step 1. Patient Positioning
- Place the patient in the lateral decubitus position.
- Support the arm with an airplane splint (Figure 29-1).

Step 2. Incisions
- Incision 1: Place a 5-mm trocar and 30-degree thoracoscope through the fifth or sixth intercostal space in the mid-axillary line (Figure 29-2).
- Incision 2: Make a 2-cm incision over the third rib in the mid-axillary line.

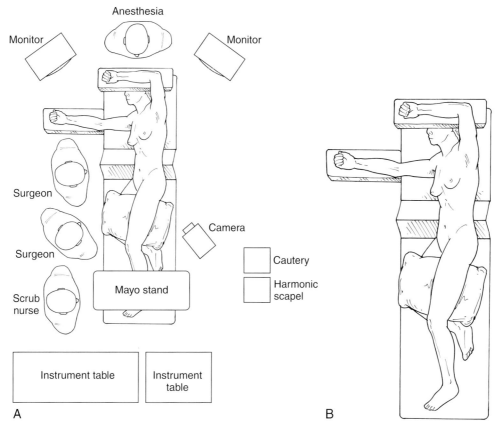

Figure 29-1. **A** and **B**, Positioning of the patient for video-assisted first rib resection. (Modified from Wolf RK, Crawford AH, Hahn B: Thoracoscopic first rib resection for thoracic outlet syndrome. In Yim APC, Hazelrigg SR, Izzat MB, et al (eds): *Minimal access cardiothoracic surgery*, Philadelphia, Saunders, 2000, pp. 330-331, Figs. 41-2 and 41-3.)

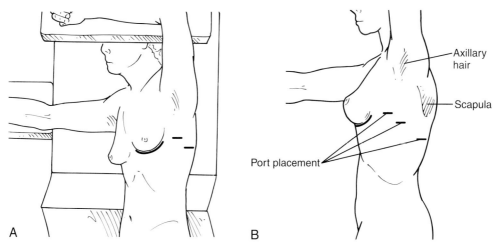

Figure 29-2. **A** and **B**, Incisions for video-assisted first rib resection. (Modified from Wolf RK, Crawford AH, Hahn B: Thoracoscopic first rib resection for thoracic outlet syndrome. In Yim APC, Hazelrigg SR, Izzat MB, et al (eds): *Minimal access cardiothoracic surgery*, Philadelphia, Saunders, 2000, p. 331.)

Step 3. Identification of the First Rib

+ **Exposure:** Decompresses the lung with carbon dioxide insufflation.
+ Aim the thoracoscope anteriorly with the 30-degree lens pointed apically.
+ Identify the first rib (Figure 29-3). The vessels can be seen in the cupola above the first rib.
+ Dissect the parietal pleura and intercostal muscles from the costal edge of the first rib using the Harmonic scalpel (Ethicon Endosurgery, Cincinnati, Ohio) (Figure 29-4).
+ The Harmonic scalpel, which operates with ultrasonic energy and produces less smoke and lower heat than regular electrocautery, is used to facilitate endoscopic dissection of the first rib.[2]
+ Bluntly dissect to the surface of the ribs and then caudally to the first rib, which is identified by feeling the flat, unique conformation of the rib.
+ Confirm identification of the first rib visually with the thoracoscope. The subclavian artery can be seen on the superior aspect of the rib.

Step 4. Dissection of the First Rib

+ **Exposure:** Use carbon dioxide insufflation.
+ Aim the thoracoscope anteriorly with the 30-degree lens pointed apically.
+ Bluntly dissect the lateral surface of the first rib with a periosteal elevator.
+ Bluntly dissect the superior surface of the first rib with a periosteal elevator.
+ Pass a right-angle clamp over the top of the first rib.
+ The subclavian vein, subclavian artery, and brachial plexus, lying from anterior to posterior and draped over the first rib, are bluntly freed using an endoscopic Cobb elevator and endoscopic curettes.
+ Cautious dissection with a transverse process elevator frees the rib circumferentially.
+ Protect the neurovascular bundle with the index finger that goes through the incision and parallel to the elevator. Keep the finger between the elevator and the neurovascular bundle to minimize the chance of damaging those structures.
+ Bluntly dissect the inferior surface of the first rib with a periosteal elevator. Stay extrapleurally because the carbon dioxide decompression of the lung is lost after opening the pleura, and the operative field is ecchymotic after the pleura is opened.
+ Pass a right-angle clamp around the superior aspect of the rib (Figure 29-5).
+ Remove a 1-cm piece of the first rib in the mid-axillary line (Figure 29-6). This allows the surgeon to push the rib caudally to complete the mobilization to the sternum (anteriorly) and the vertebral bodies (posteriorly).

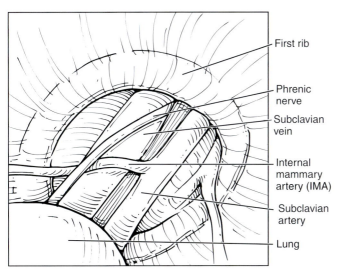

First rib

Phrenic nerve

Subclavian vein

Internal mammary artery (IMA)

Subclavian artery

Lung

Figure 29-3. Identification of the first rib. (Modified from Wolf RK, Crawford AH, Hahn B: Thoracoscopic first rib resection for thoracic outlet syndrome. In Yim APC, Hazelrigg SR, Izzat MB, et al (eds): *Minimal access cardiothoracic surgery*, Philadelphia, Saunders, 2000, p. 332.)

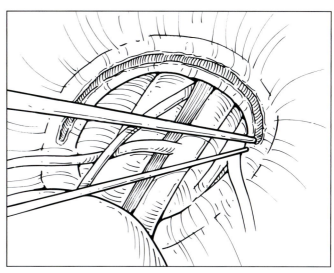

Figure 29-4. Harmonic scalpel mobilization of pleura and muscles for the first rib resection. (Modified from Wolf RK, Crawford AH, Hahn B: Thoracoscopic first rib resection for thoracic outlet syndrome. In Yim APC, Hazelrigg SR, Izzat MB, et al (eds): *Minimal access cardiothoracic surgery*, Philadelphia, WB Saunders, 2000, p. 332.)

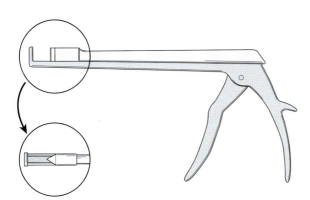

Figure 29-5. Rib cutter (Sofamor Danek, Nashville, TN). (Modified from Wolf RK, Crawford AH, Hahn B: Thoracoscopic first rib resection for thoracic outlet syndrome. Yim APC, Hazelrigg SR, Izzat MB, et al (eds): *Minimal access cardiothoracic surgery*, Philadelphia, Saunders, 2000, p. 333.)

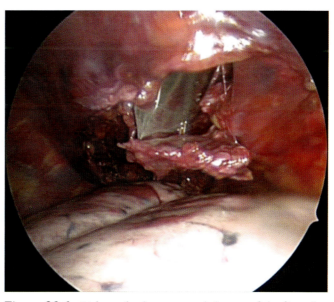

Figure 29-6. Right-angle clamp around the top of the first rib.

- ◆ Cut the rib with a rib cutter (Figure 29-7).
- ◆ After transection of the rib, any additional muscle attachments, such as the scalenus anticus or medius, can be divided under direct vision.
- ◆ Remove the pieces of the rib. The rib can be delivered easily through one of the port sites after removing the port.
- ◆ After complete thoracoscopic first rib excision, the contents of the neurovascular bundle drape gently across the apex of the pleural cavity. The extent of rib resection and its immediate effect on the structures of the thoracic outlet are clearly visualized (Figure 29-8).

References

1. Poole GV, Thomae KR: Thoracic outlet syndrome reconsidered, *Am Surg* 62:287–291, 1996.
2. Ohtsuka T, Wolf RK, Dunsker SB: Port-access first-rib resection, *Surg Endosc* 13:940–942, 1999.
3. Yim APC, Hazelrigg SR, Izzat MB, et al (eds): Minimal access cardiothoracic surgery, Pheladelphia, Saunders, 2000.

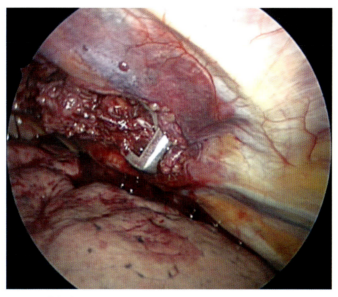

Figure 29-7. Cutting the rib by the vertebral body.

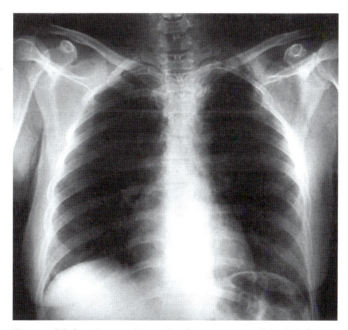

Figure 29-8. Chest radiograph after resection of the left first rib. (From Wolf RK, Crawford AH, Hahn B: Thoracoscopic first rib resection for thoracic outlet syndrome. In Yim APC, Hazelrigg SR, Izzat MB, et al (eds): *Minimal access cardiothoracic surgery,* Philadelphia, Saunders, 2000, p. 334.)

CHAPTER 30

MINIMALLY INVASIVE SURGERY FOR ATRIAL FIBRILLATION

Randall Kevin Wolf and Eric W. Schneeberger

Introduction

During the past decade, surgeons' experience with video-assisted thoracic surgical (VATS) approaches has increased, and technologic advances in minimally invasive instrumentation have been made. One result of these improvements is that surgical ablation for atrial fibrillation can be successfully performed using minimally invasive techniques.

Approach to Video-Assisted Thoracic Surgery for Atrial Fibrillation

Order of Operative Steps

The order of the steps of the operation is as follows: establish working ports, open the pericardium, perform baseline electrophysiologic testing (including ganglion plexus stimulation), encircle pulmonary veins, isolate pulmonary veins, perform directed partial denervation of the heart, and remove the left atrial appendage (LAA).

Key Points

- Patients who choose a minimally invasive surgical approach to correcting atrial fibrillation usually are otherwise in good health. There is no room for error, and the mortality rate must be zero.
- Our bilateral VATS technique is designed to allow cardiac surgeons to achieve atrial fibrillation cures safely but without mastering totally thoracoscopic skills.
- The bilateral working ports are deliberately positioned directly over the pulmonary veins and on the left side over the LAA to allow direct (three-dimensional) visualization of these important structures. This increases the safety margin, especially for less experienced surgeons.

Video-Assisted Surgery for Atrial Fibrillation

Step 1. Setup

- Use a double-lumen endotracheal tube for selective lung ventilation, and place the central line, arterial line, and external defibrillator pads in the appropriate vector.
- Use sequential compression stockings on the lower extremities and a warmer to control body temperature.

Step 2. Patient Positioning and Port Placement

- Place the patient in the left lateral decubitus position at 45 to 60 degrees, with the right arm on an LPS Arm Support (Allen Medical, Acton, Maine).
- Document the external anatomy after reviewing the internal anatomy using the chest radiograph. Outline the scapula, mid-axillary line, and a line from the xyphoid posteriorly (Figure 30-1).
- Make the incisions as shown in Figure 30-2.
- First port placement
  - ▲ Place the first port in the sixth or seventh intercostal space in the mid-axillary line where the xyphoid line and mid-axillary lines cross.
  - ▲ Place the thoracoscope with a 30-degree lens in this port.
- Large working port placement
  - ▲ Through the thoracoscope, identify the third (or fourth) intercostal space.
  - ▲ Make a 4- to 6-cm working incision from the auscultatory triangle in the third or fourth intercostal space, and carry it anteriorly.
  - ▲ For the muscle-sparing technique, if the third intercostal space is used, only the intercostal muscles need to be divided. If the fourth intercostal space is used, divide the serratus anterior in the direction of the muscle fibers. Avoid cutting the pectoralis muscle by retracting it anteriorly (Figure 30-3).
  - ▲ Use caution posteriorly to retract the fat pad containing any neurovascular bundle with a finger when carrying the incision over the axillary contents.
  - ▲ Insert a medium CardioVations soft tissue retractor (Edwards Lifesciences, Irvine, Calif) through the large working port.

Step 3. Pericardial Opening

- **Exposure:** Retract the lung directly posteriorly.
- Aim the thoracoscope anteriorly with the 30-degree lens pointed posteromedially.
- Turn the electrocautery down to 15 or 20 watts.
- Open the pericardium a few centimeters anterior and parallel to the right phrenic nerve; a plastic sucker may be used to insulate the heart from the electrocautery (Figure 30-4).
- Visualize the phrenic nerve during pericardial opening and throughout the procedure to avoid contact, traction, compression, or electrocautery injury to the phrenic nerve.
- Place one or two pericardial stay sutures in the lateral-cut pericardial edge, and anchor them as far posteriorly as possible with CardioVations suture snares through separate stab sites. Place a superior pericardial stay suture adjacent to the superior vena cava and right pulmonary artery to improve direct visualization and access.
- Place an inferior pericardial stay suture adjacent to the inferior aspect of the inferior pulmonary artery to provide optimal access for opening the oblique sinus. If necessary, place an additional stay suture adjacent to the bifurcation of the right pulmonary veins.
- At this stage, verify adequate visualization directly through the incision and endoscope. Ensure that all of the relevant anatomic (superior vena cava, right superior pulmonary vein, right inferior pulmonary vein, inferior vena cava, and right pulmonary artery) structures can be clearly visualized.

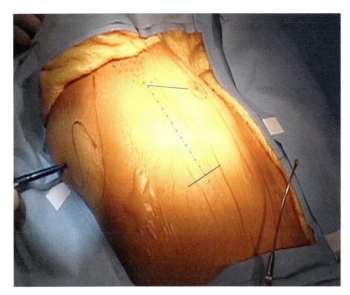

Figure 30-1. Anatomic landmarks used to position the incisions properly.

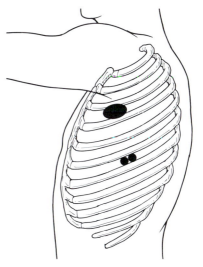

Figure 30-2. Incisions used for video-assisted thoracic surgery for atrial fibrillation.

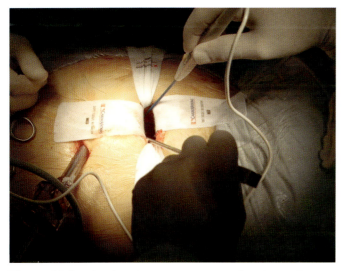

Figure 30-3. The skin retractor is positioned in the working incision.

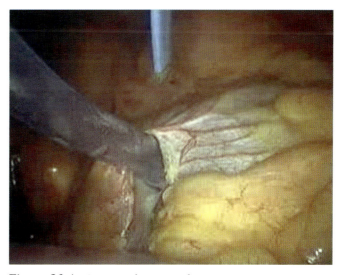

Figure 30-4. Opening the pericardium.

Step 4. Encircling the Pulmonary Veins

*   **Exposure:** Retract the lung posteriorly, and retract the heart medially.
*   Aim the thoracoscope anteriorly with the 30-degree lens pointed posteriorly.
*   With a pediatric long Wolf or Yankauer suction (Scanlan International, St. Paul, Minn), bluntly develop a space just inferior to the inferior pulmonary vein and lateral to the inferior vena cava into the oblique sinus. Confirm that the suction device can fall freely into the oblique sinus through this opening.
*   Use the endoscope to check the access angle for the Wolf Lumitip dissector (AtriCure, West Chester, Ohio). A sponge stick can be used to gently retract the heart medially as needed for access and visualization.
*   Create a second working port (10 mm) 5 cm medially or laterally to the endoscope port for dissector use. This allows the dissector to be lined up for direct in-line access with the appropriate port.
*   The GlidePath (AtriCure) is attached to the dissector by inserting the dissector tip into the GlidePath hood (Figure 30-5). The Wolf Lumitip dissector with GlidePath is introduced with no articulation through the port site into the pericardial space. Use caution not to direct the tip of the dissector toward the heart when introduced.
*   Bluntly retract the superior vena cava medially with an endoscopic kittner to help gain exposure and visualization of the superior aspect of the right pulmonary artery. Feed the dissector tip into the oblique sinus just above the inferior vena cava (see Figure 30-5). Advance the distal end of the dissector tip posteriorly, and sweep it medially into position behind the right pulmonary veins, articulate the lighted dissector and grasp the plastic GlidePath and remove the Wolf dissector.

Step 5. Baseline Electrophysiology Testing

*   **Exposure:** Retract the heart medially with a sponge stick.
*   Aim the thoracoscope anteriorly with the 30-degree lens pointed posteriorly.
*   Use the AtriCure pen and the AtriCure ORLab (Figure 30-6) to document sensing over the right atrium and the pulmonary veins.
*   If the heart is in sinus rhythm, pacing also can be documented.
*   With the AtriCure pen, perform high-frequency stimulation of the fat pad areas over Waterston's groove. They are stimulated in a grid pattern (Figure 30-7) with the AtriCure system (Figure 30-8).
*   Record sites where a vagal response is elicited.

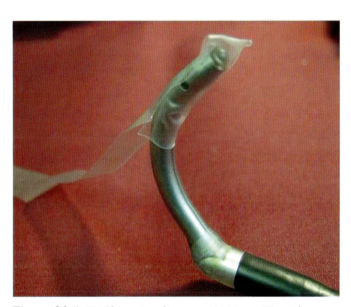

Figure 30-5. Wolf Lumitip dissector (AtriCure, West Chester, Ohio) with the AtriCure GlidePath hood.

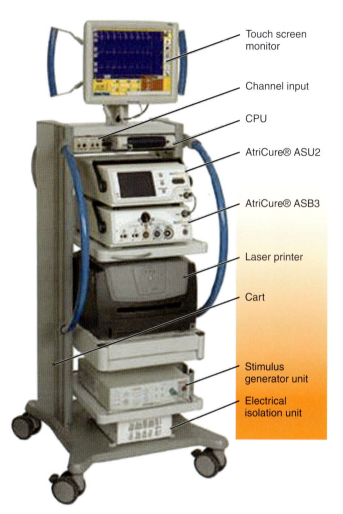

Figure 30-6. AtriCure's ORLab system.

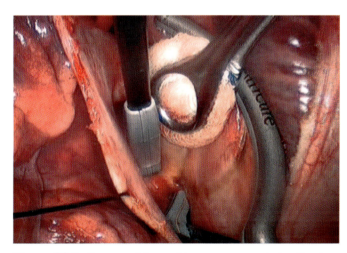

Figure 30-7. Sponge stick provides exposure and visualization of the superior aspect of the right pulmonary artery.

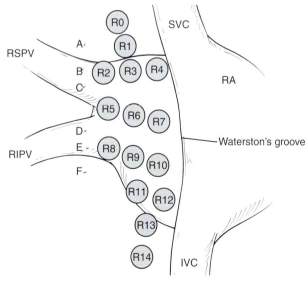

Figure 30-8. Fat pad areas over Waterston's groove are stimulated in a grid pattern. *IVC,* inferior vena cava; *RA,* right atrium; *RIPV,* right inferior pulmonary vein; *RSPV,* right superior pulmonary vein; *SVC,* superior vena cava.

Step 6. Isolating the Pulmonary Veins

- **Exposure:** Retract the heart medially.
- Aim the thoracoscope anteriorly with the 30-degree lens pointed posteriorly.
- Advance the lower jaw of the Isolator (AtriCure) clamp into the oblique sinus. Advance the Isolator lower jaw until its posterior tip is visible superior to the superior pulmonary vein, making sure to apply adequate tension to the red rubber catheter to help lead the lower jaw into place (Figure 30-9).
- Create transmural and contiguous lesions on the antrum to electrically isolate the pulmonary veins from the remainder of the heart.
- After completing the ablation, place the AtriCure pen on the previously recorded locations of the superior pulmonary vein, inferior pulmonary vein, and the bifurcation of the right ventricles. Record the electrocardiogram (ECG).
- If the ECG recording shows quiescence in all locations on the pulmonary veins where A waves or P waves (if the heart is in sinus rhythm) had been seen before the ablation, the pulmonary vein isolation is complete. If the heart is in sinus rhythm, pacing also can be checked.

Step 7. Directed Partial Denervation of the Heart

- **Exposure:** Retract the lung directly posteriorly, and retract the heart medially with a sponge stick.
- Aim the thoracoscope anteriorly with the 30-degree lens pointed posteriorly.
- The bipolar pen is used to ablate active fat pad areas of the ganglionated plexuses.

Step 8. Closure

- Place bipolar temporary pacing leads under the medial cut edge of the pericardium. The pressure of the pericardium ensures contact with the right atrium without the need to suture the leads to the epicardium.
- Bring this lead through one of the inferior ports.
- Bring a Blake chest tube out through one of the inferior ports.
- Perform intercostal blocks for ribs 3 through 6.
- Place On-Q catheters percutaneously, and with thoracoscopic assistance, tunnel one catheter just outside the parietal pleura in the working port interspace. The second catheter is placed through the working port incision.

Video-Assisted Surgery for Atrial Fibrillation on the Left Side

Step 1. Patient Positioning and Access

- The positioning, access ports, and exposure are identical to those on the right side.
- The dissection and ablation are performed similar to the procedure on the right side, except on the left side, the ligament of Marshall must be divided.

Step 2. Ligament of Marshall

- **Exposure:** Retract the left pulmonary artery superiorly and the LAA medially.
- Aim the thoracoscope anteriorly with the 30-degree lens pointed posteriorly.
- The ligament of Marshall is the remnant of the embryologic left superior vena cava, and it runs from the underside of the left pulmonary artery to the roof of the left atrium (Figure 30-10).
- Use electrocautery with care to prevent damage to the left pulmonary artery or left atrium.
- On the left side, there is nothing below the left inferior pulmonary vein. The dissector is introduced below the vein and directed to emerge medial to the divided ligament of Marshall (Figure 30-11).

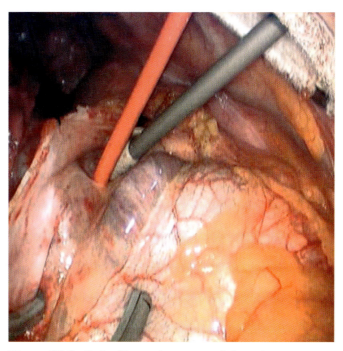

Figure 30-9. Red rubber catheter around the atrium.

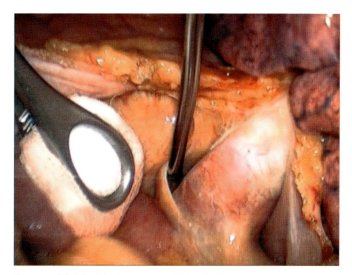

Figure 30-10. The ligament of Marshall.

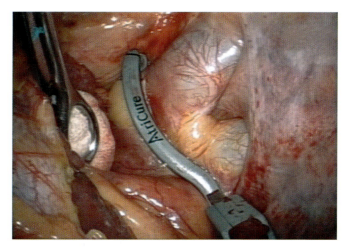

Figure 30-11. Placement of the AtriCure pen on the left side.

Step 3. Removal of the Left Atrial Appendage

- Retract the pericardium anteriorly with one pericardial stay suture.
- Aim the thoracoscope anteriorly with the 30-degree lens pointed posteriorly.
- After the left pulmonary veins have been isolated, exclude the LAA.
- Use an EZ 45 stapler (Ethicon Endosurgery, Cincinnati, Ohio) with a thick tissue load (e.g., green load, staple height of 4.8 mm) to excise the LAA (Figure 30-12).
- The stapler should be introduced through the most posteriorly located inferior port site.
- The stapler must be advanced in the groove between the appendage and the heart with the tip of the stapler positioned underneath the pulmonary artery.
- The stapler is fired across the base of the LAA to excise the entire LAA.

Step 4. Closing the Pericardium

- Close the pericardium on the left side to avoid herniation of the heart. Use the stay sutures or additional sutures to close the pericardium.
- The remainder of the closure on the left side is similar to that for the right side (Figure 30-13).
- Patients are routinely extubated in the operating suite.

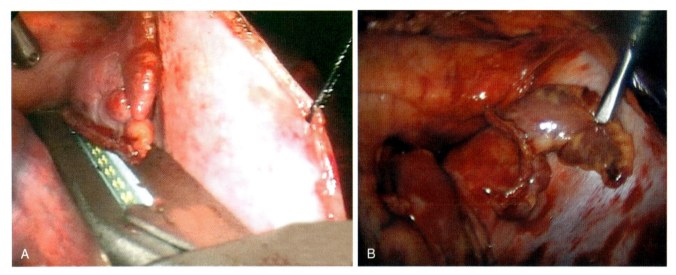

Figure 30-12. **A** and **B,** The endoscopic stapler is used to excise the left atrial appendage.

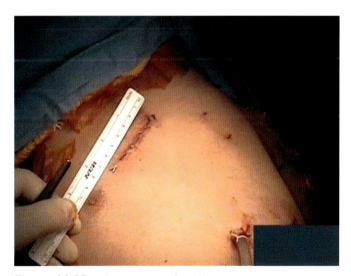

Figure 30-13. The incisions after closure.

CHAPTER 31

THORACOSCOPIC APPROACH TO SPINAL DEFORMITIES

Randall Kevin Wolf and A. Atiq Durrani

Introduction

The conventional approaches to the spine have been posterolateral, costotransverse, and anterior. To reach the anterior spine, anterior thoracotomy has traditionally been used. Problems associated with thoracotomy include a long incision, rib resection, significant rib spreading, tissue desiccation, alteration of pulmonary and shoulder girdle function, significant pain, associated morbidity, and poor cosmesis. The field of video-assisted thoracic surgery (VATS) presents the spinal surgeon with an endoscopic option for approaching the anterior vertebral column.

The use of video-assisted thoracoscopy can decrease the surgical morbidity associated with open procedures. The goals and objectives of this newer technique are the same as those for thoracotomy. The VATS approach to the spine has led to many exciting new techniques for treatment of the disk space. Surgical instruments, guided by an endoscope, are able to gain access to the chest through 15- to 20-mm ports rather than through the 8- to 10-inch-long incision required for thoracotomy.

In December 1993, at Children's Hospital Medical Center in Cincinnati, we began performing VATS for the anterior release of severe spinal deformities in children and adolescents. The benefits of this procedure include minimal invasiveness, better visualization and magnification, diminished postoperative pain and ventilatory compromise, reduced blood loss, decreased hospitalization, reduced health-care costs, improved wound care, and earlier return to prehospital activities with minimal shoulder dysfunction.[1]

Indications for Children and Adolescents

- Rigid idiopathic scoliosis deformities at or above 75 degrees in magnitude with correction to less than 50 degrees seen on side-bending radiographs
- Prevention of crankshaft phenomenon in the skeletally immature child who has more than a 50-degree curvature
- Kyphotic deformities greater than 70 degrees
- Neuromuscular deformities accompanied by at-risk pulmonary status
- Progressive spinal deformity and metabolic disease
- Severe rib hump deformity not corrected by spinal instrumentation
- Neurofibromatosis with intrathoracic tumors in addition to a significant spinal deformity
- Pseudarthrosis after anterior intervertebral fusion
- Anterior hemiepiphysiodesis for congenital scoliosis
- Incision and excision biopsy

    We have extended our indications to include all the procedures addressing the thoracic spine that were previously approached by thoracotomy.[2]

Approach to Minimally Invasive Exposure of the Thoracic Spine

Order of Operative Steps

The order of steps of the operation is as follows: confirm somatosensory evoked potential (SSEP) monitoring, place the patient in the prone position, mark the topical anatomy under fluoroscopic control, establish ports, expose the appropriate disk levels, and provide exposure for disk removal or for stapling.

Key Points

- Working ports should be placed in order to align the instruments fairly straight into the disk spaces.
- At least three ports are recommended. One port is needed for a pediatric Wolf or Yankauer suction (Scanlon International, St. Paul, Minn). One port is used for the thoracoscope. This leaves one working port. An additional lower port or incision is used for the Endokittner (Ethicon Endosurgery, Cincinnati, Ohio) to depress the diaphragm. By shifting the instruments from port to port, T2 to L1 can be instrumented (Figure 31-1).
- The Harmonic scalpel is used to open the parietal pleura and, when indicated, to divide the intercostal vessels.
- The endoscopic hardware includes various angled thoracoscopes capable of magnifying up to 15 times, as well as specialized thoracospinal instruments (e.g., rongeurs, curettes, periosteal elevators, electrocautery, Harmonic scalpel, and suction irrigation devices).[3]

Video-Assisted Thoracic Spinal Surgery

Step 1. Setup and Patient Positioning

- Initiate routine intraoperative monitoring for thoracic procedures (e.g., arterial pressure line) and somatosensory evoked potential (SSEP) monitoring.
- Administer general anesthesia through a double-lumen endotracheal tube or bronchial blocker.
- Turn the patient to the prone position.

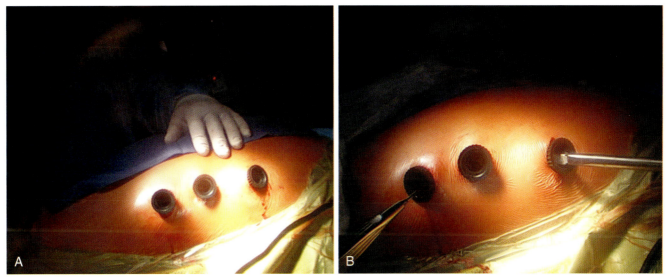

Figure 31-1. **A,** Typical ports for thoracic spine exposure. **B,** The thoracoscope usually is in the middle port, and instruments are placed in the superior and inferior ports.

Step 2. Establishing Working Ports

- Because curves are usually convex to the right, the surgeon usually stands on the patient's right side. However, the approach, based on the curve, should be confirmed with the surgeon before placing the patient on the operating table.
- The topographic anatomy, specifically the scapular borders, the twelfth rib, and the iliac crest, are identified and outlined with a marker. If simultaneous posterior approach is used, confirm the levels by fluoroscopy.
- Three to five portals usually are necessary. The first portal is most frequently placed at or about the T6 or T7 interspace in the posterior axillary line. Entry at this level usually avoids the diaphragm.
- Insufflation in the thoracic cavity is not necessary because of the rigidity of the chest wall and the ability to collapse the ipsilateral lung. Open trocars are used, and a variety of disposable trocars are available (e.g., Ethicon Endosurgery).
- Use a 15-mm simple trocar, through which a 10-mm, 30-degree, rigid telescope is placed. We use rigid and flexible ports (Ethicon Endosurgery) for positioning and inserting instruments.
- If posterior spinal instrumentation is being performed, the posterior approach is started simultaneously by the surgeon, who usually is positioned on the left side (Figure 31-2).

Step 3. Visualization and Assessment

- The 30-degree thoracoscope allows direct vision into the intervertebral disk spaces without impeding the surgical instrumentation or obscuring the operative field.
- The instruments can be switched from portal to portal, keeping the working portal aligned straight with the area of interest, usually the disk.
- The camera and viewing field are rotated 90 degrees from the standard VATS position, because the spinal surgeon is most comfortable viewing and approaching the spine through a horizontal projection.
- Carry out a panoramic assessment and evaluation of the intrathoracic space to determine the anatomy and possible sites for other ports that allow a more direct working approach to the intervertebral disks. The ports are usually two interspaces apart (see Figure 31-1B).
- Visualize the superior thoracic spine without retraction after the lung is completely deflated.
- Retraction of the diaphragm is necessary below T7 to L1. An endokittner works well for this maneuver.
- The primary and other working portal sites are selected by this method.
- After the spinal anatomy has been identified, select the levels for performing annulotomy and diskectomy. The ribs are counted by visualization and confirmed by fluoroscopy. Insert a wire into an intervertebral disk, and obtain a radiograph.
- The superior intercostal vein usually empties into the azygous circulation at or about the T3 or T4 interspace. Approach the vertebral column through the parietal pleura.[4]

Step 4. Opening the Parietal Pleura

- Use a dissecting hook Harmonic scalpel (Ethicon Endosurgery) for opening the parietal pleura (Figure 31-3).
- Identify the intervertebral disk by the mounds observed on the spinal column and the vertebral bodies by the valleys. The segmental vessels nest in the valleys directly overlying the bodies (see Figure 31-3).
- Multilevel anterior diskectomies are necessary for correcting severe spinal deformity. This anterior release of the spinal curvature usually requires diskectomy at six to eight levels. For degenerative disease, fewer levels are targeted.
- Elevate the pleura, and retract it with thoracoscopic periosteal elevators and blunt dissectors. With the Harmonic scalpel, coagulate any vessels that appear to be at risk for bleeding.

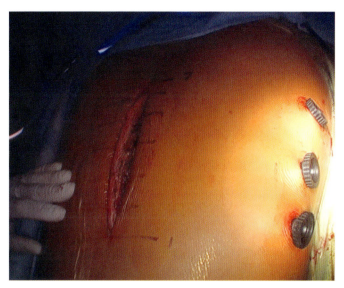

Figure 31-2. Simultaneous posterior approach and placement of the ports.

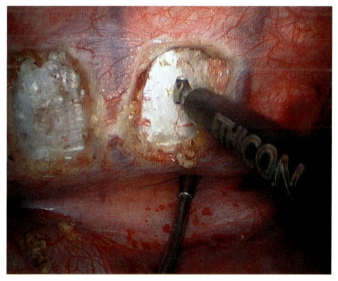

Figure 31-3. The Harmonic scalpel is used to open the parietal pleura.

Step 5. Excision of the Thoracic Disk

- After the pleura has been completely dissected at the appropriate levels, proceed directly to excision of the annulus at the level of the intervertebral disk. Use a technique that is comfortable.
- The assistant surgeon keeps vessels retracted from another port using a long Wolf pediatric or Yankauer suction.
- Make a transverse cut across the vertebral body, anterior to the rib heads, and parallel to the disk that is rostral and caudal to it.
- Use an elevator for lifting the periosteum toward the vertebral endplate and isolating the disk.
- Make a transverse cut across the annulus fibrosus, and continue down to the level of the nucleus pulposus. Use rongeurs, curettes, periosteal elevators, and high-rpm protected drills as necessary to ensure complete removal of the disk material and the endplates (Figure 31-4).
- The length of the rongeurs' jaws should be measured to the hinge so that the depth of penetration toward the posterior longitudinal ligament can be determined. In a young child, it is often possible to elevate the vertebral endplate apophysis and completely excise the intervertebral contents back to the posterior longitudinal ligament.
- With experience, the surgeon improves the ability to excise the annulus and disk space contents in an approximately 250-degree arc, or almost from pedicle to pedicle. Direct particular attention to the release of the annulus on the concave side (Figure 31-5).
- Stress the spinal column segment by rotating the periosteal elevator in the disk space and exercising moderate force after each release to determine whether mobility has been achieved. Bone cages usually are placed into disk spaces (Figure 31-6). Insert a small piece of Gelfoam or Surgicel around the cage (Figure 31-7).
- After completion of the procedure, remove all disk fragments and debris from the thoracic cavity; the pleura remains open (Figure 31-8).
- Connect a chest tube to the water seal.
- During the procedure, the greater splanchnic nerve is usually transected at one of several levels. This does not cause permanent residual problems, but parents and the pediatric patient should understand that there is a possibility of a hot and cold "sympathetic release" phenomenon on the contralateral or ipsilateral lower extremity after this kind of surgery. This phenomenon is similar to what is experienced after a transthoracic thoracotomy is performed.

References

1. Crawford AH, Wolf RK: Spinal deformities. In Yim AP, Hazler SR, Izzat MB, et al, editors: *Minimal access cardiothoracic surgery*, Philadelphia, 2000, Saunders, pp. 316–327.
2. Crawford AH, Wolf RK, Wall EJ, et al: Pediatric spinal deformity. In Regan JJ, McAfee PC, Mack MJ, editors: *Atlas of endoscopic spine surgery*, St Louis, 1995, Quality Medical Publishing.
3. Crawford AH: Video-assisted thoracoscopy. In *Spine: State of the Art Reviews II*, Philadelphia, 1997, Hanely & Belfus.
4. Mack MJ, Regan JJ, McFee PC, et al: Video-assisted thoracic surgery for the anterior approach to the thoracic spine, *Ann Thorac Surg* 59:1102–1106, 1995.

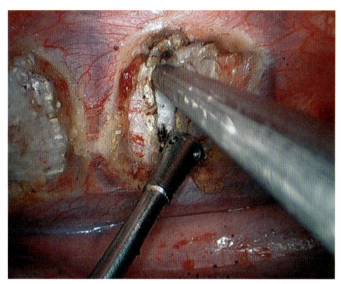

Figure 31-4. The drill is used to remove the disk material and the endplates.

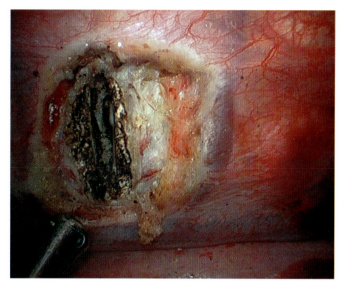

Figure 31-5. Empty disk space.

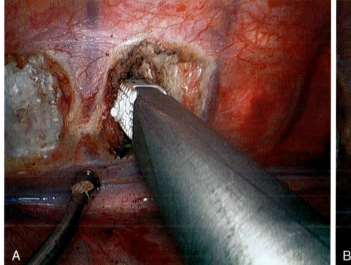

Figure 31-6. **A** and **B,** A bone cage is placed into the disk space.

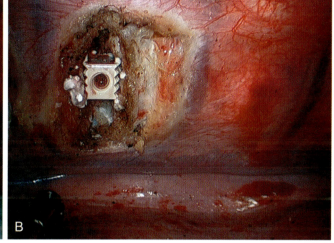

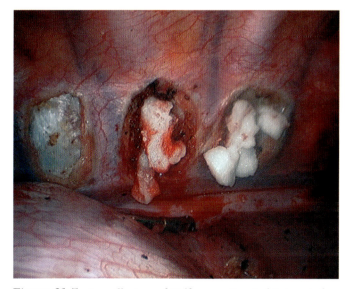

Figure 31-7. A small piece of Gelfoam or Surgicel is inserted around the cage.

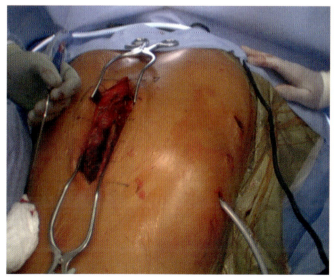

Figure 31-8. Simultaneous posterior and right lateral approaches with the patient in the prone position.

CHAPTER 32

DIAPHRAGMATIC PLICATION —

VIDEO 32

Robert J. McKenna, Jr.

Introduction

Plication of a paralyzed diaphragm can relieve dyspnea and substantially improve pulmonary function. The procedure is underused and may be performed well as video-assisted thoracic surgery (VATS). The diaphragm absorbs the pleural fluid created daily in the pleural space, and when the diaphragm is plicated well, there is much less absorptive surface. Patients may drain a surprisingly large amount of fluid postoperatively through the chest tube, and the hospital stay may be 1 week.

Approach to Video-Assisted Diaphragmatic Plication

Order of Operative Steps

The order of the steps of the operation is as follows: caudal pressure on the diaphragm and repeated suturing of the diaphragm obliquely from anterior to posterior (Video 32-1).

Key Points

- The chronically paralyzed diaphragm is displaced very superiorly.
- Good exposure is the key to starting the procedure. The incision in the auscultatory triangle produces downward pressure on the diaphragm to provide exposure for the procedure.
- The plication is performed anteromedially to posterolaterally, with running sutures placed back and forth.
- Make the incisions low enough so the diaphragm may be plicated tightly.

Video-Assisted Diaphragmatic Plication

Step 1. Incisions

- **Exposure:** The procedure is usually performed through three incisions (Figure 32-1) (see Video 32-1).
- Incision 1: Make a 2-cm incision in the mid-clavicular line in about the sixth intercostal space. This is usually one space below the mammary crease. This incision is used for suturing the diaphragm.
- Incision 2: Make a 1-cm incision (used for the trocar and thoracoscope) in the mid-axillary line in the eighth intercostal space. Although we normally use a short reusable trocar for this procedure, we typically use a longer disposable trocar because the diaphragm touches the lens until it is pushed caudally and plicated. Initially, the incision seems too low because the diaphragm is so high, but the low positioning of the thoracoscope helps in creating a very tight plication with maximal downward displacement of the paralyzed diaphragm.
- Incision 3: Make a 1-cm incision in the auscultatory space. This is usually 4 finger-breadths below the tip of the scapula and halfway toward the spine. This incision is used to apply downward pressure on the diaphragm.

Step 2. Pressure on the Diaphragm

- **Exposure:** Push the diaphragm caudally.
- Aim the thoracoscope toward the apex of the chest with the 30-degree lens pointed anteriorly.
- Through the incision in the auscultatory incision, apply downward pressure with a ring forceps on the diaphragm (Figure 32-2).

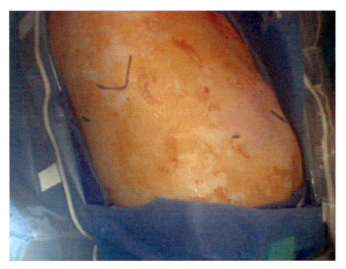

Figure 32-1. Incisions used to plicate the diaphragm.

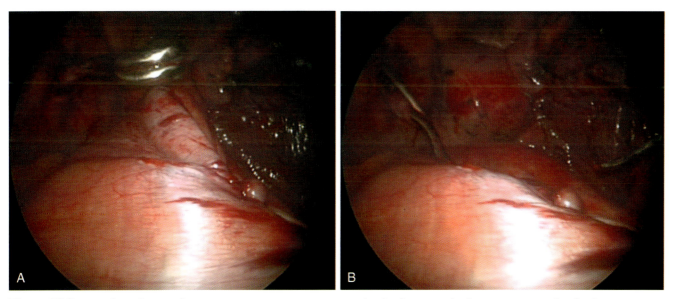

Figure 32-2. **A** and **B,** The ring forceps are in position to compress the diaphragm and, after compressing the diaphragm, to facilitate the plication.

Step 3. Plication of the Diaphragm

- **Exposure:** Push the diaphragm caudally.
- Aim the thoracoscope apically with the 30-degree lens pointed anteriorly.
- Pass a needle driver with 0 Prolene suture or the Endostitch (Covidien, Norwalk, Conn) through the mid-clavicular line to start the plication anteriorly (Figure 32-3).
- The ring forceps from a posterior direction indents the diaphragm for the plication.
- Suturing proceeds anteromedially to posterolaterally. The suture grabs a 1-cm purchase of the diaphragm on both sides of the indented diaphragm. Tie the suture extracorporeally, and pull the tail through incision 1. Retract the tail of the suture to help with exposure.
- The initial sutures are the most difficult to place because the space is small.
- As the plication proceeds, compress areas of the diaphragm with a ring forceps from a posterior direction. Multiple layers of suture are placed so the first layer creates a small plication.
- The suture is run anteriorly to posteriorly and then back anteriorly to be tied to the tail of the suture.
- The plications continue until the diaphragm is very tight (Figure 32-4).

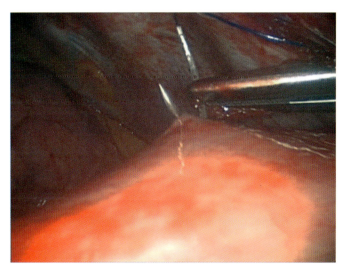

Figure 32-3. The needle driver is inserted through the anteroinferior incision to start the plication anteriorly.

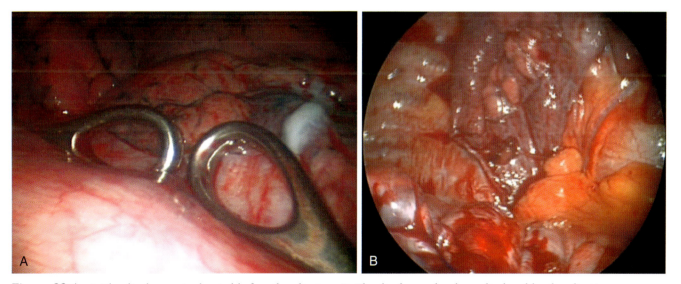

Figure 32-4. A, The diaphragm is elevated before the plication. **B,** The diaphragm has been displaced by the plication.

INDEX

Note: Page numbers followed by *f* indicate figures and *t* indicate tables.